BODY CONSCIOUS

BODY CONSCIOUS

A WOMAN'S GUIDE TO HOLISTIC PELVIC WELLNESS AND FEMININE EMBODIMENT

TARYN GAUDIN

DRAWINGS BY LARA HARDY - BILLIE HARDY
CREATIVE

TARYN GAUDIN

CONTENTS

First Printing, 2021

1

WELCOME

INVITING EMPOWERED RESPONSIBILITY

Within this book, I share both clinical evidence-based information, alongside my understanding of energy medicine. Before you read on I invite you to take empowered responsibility for your health and wellbeing. Whilst there is a depth of information within the pages of this book, you maintain autonomous ownership of your health. What I offer within Body Conscious is *not* personalised medical advice, and in no way replaces personalised medical/health advice. My vision is that you take the pieces of this book that feel resonate and true for you, and use these pieces alongside any guidance that you choose to seek from your health care and medical professionals.

MY STORY

Six weeks after giving birth I started running again. Fourteen months later I was representing Australia at The Triathlon Age Group World Championships in Chicago. Even though I was a first-time mother and tired as hell with a baby who didn't sleep, I got there through the determination, discipline, and dedication that had seen me a national-level gymnast at 12 years of age. Since retiring from gymnastics I was an avid gym-goer, a marathon runner, an ocean swimmer, a cyclist, and a Pilates and Yoga enthusiast. Being fit, and keeping my body toned was more than just a hobby, it was almost an obsession. Just months after giving birth I felt strong, fit, and fast. I was proud of what my body could *do*, and for a fleeting moment, I was happy with how my body looked. But soon enough the strong self-criticism and self-evaluation returned. But I didn't want to go back to that place, I was determined not to.

The birth of my first child was a strong catalyst that caused me to stop and look at my life and my relationship with myself and my body. I had a burning desire to create a lifestyle that felt more like me, in particular, I had this exciting, yet irritating, sensation that I was capable of creating a career that was more meaningful and rewarding. My work as a hospital physiotherapist didn't feel fulfilling, and even though I reached a senior position relatively early in my career, I wasn't excited to return to it. Being at home with my family was most important to me, and I knew that if I was sacrificing time with my family, I wanted to be doing something that lit me up from within. These sensations propelled me on an uncomfortable and overwhelming journey. I had so many questions. What is my purpose? What is the work that I will love? What do I want my life to look like? What would make me feel good more often? I knew I wanted to work with women, but I had no idea in what capacity. I knew I wanted flexibility in my work, but had no idea what that would look like. I knew I wanted that fleeting feeling of body peace, and that embodied sensation of knowing the strength, power, and possibility of being in a woman's body to last, but HOW? It was here that I became curious about my life and my inner landscape, but it wasn't until I had had my second child that I felt like I fully committed to the path of self-discovery.

The birth of my second child and the persistent, all-consuming pelvic pain I experienced was pivotal in helping me to create a new relationship with myself, and my body. The pain was physically and emotionally exhausting. In search of a way to fix my pain, my first point of call was to see a pelvic floor physiotherapist. I had been studying pelvic floor physiotherapy myself, and thought it would be helpful. My therapist noticed I had increased pelvic tone for which I began some relaxation exercises, self-massage, and continued with my own movement therapy. It was helpful yet the pain continued.

Alongside my physio, I saw a naturopath, took Chinese medicines, and had acupuncture therapy. The pain continued without any real improvement. Months later, I was referred to a specialist Urologist Gynaecologist. I underwent laparoscopic surgery to investigate the cause of my pain, only to find nothing.

I felt burnt-out, frustrated, and as though my body was failing me. I wasn't able to engage in the exercise I was used to, which was how I had always managed and maintained my mental health. I felt like my world was spiraling out of control. My GP prescribed antidepressants. I took them for less than three months because they made me feel so ill.

I thought I was taking a holistic approach to heal my pain and it took me a long time to realise that I wasn't. What I was doing was trying to fix my pain while I had a deep underlying sense that my body was broken. *That* was the piece that needed attention.

At the same time, I was in a state of anxiety, desperate not to return to my job at the hospital. I wanted to start my own physiotherapy clinic and work a couple of days a week, helping women to return to exercise safely after birth. Although I had become clearer about the direction I wanted my work to go in, I was trying to build a successful business quickly, doing it all blindly and on my own. Everything was on me - building a website, social media, creating online programs, continuing with study and professional development. You name it I was doing it. I was so fixated on wanting to contribute financially to our family and create a business on my own terms, whilst trying to discover my self and remain present as a moth at the same time – I know now I was attempting to do too much, in too short of time, and it wasn't sustainable.

One day I became so exhausted from trying to "fix" my pain (and my life) that I simply decided to stop fighting against my body and to try and work with it. How novel! I decided that I could continue to feel like my body was broken, and remain disconnected and disappointed, or I could work with it and finally listen to what it was trying to tell me. I could create new connections and new thought patterns about what my pain meant to me. I could embrace what movement was available to me, rather than thinking of all the things I couldn't do, and I could use my pain as a way to learn how to nourish my body.

In short, I decided to tune in and let my body lead the way, rather than trying to find a way to fix it. This was the beginning of an incredible journey where I recreated my entire relationship with myself and with my body. It would also be the pathway to finding the missing links of how I wanted to work with women, and how I could find the sense of ease I was yearning for in my work and in my life.

Once I had decided to *simply be in my body*, and let it be my guide, the layers of all the ways that I had been betraying myself, and my body, began to show. Not immediately of course, but bit by bit. With my acceptance of my pelvic pain I was able to see that even though I was a physiotherapist and had a good understanding of the human body, and even though I was an athlete and I had an acute awareness of how my body moved physically and worked functionally, there were still so many ways I forced my body to do things that were depleting my energy by pushing on even when I was utterly exhausted. I began to realise that during all of the effort, a stream of self-criticism played on repeat; a constant evaluation that always read 'not good enough'. I was tired, and my pelvic tension was my body's way of finally getting my attention.

By constantly ignoring my body's signals, not only was I denying myself the experience of being truly present in my body, I was also suppressing much of my emotional, spiritual, creative, and intuitive self. Like so many women, throughout my lifetime I had constantly ignored, criticised, and buried parts of who I am, and now in this new phase of my life, I had a deep desire to reconnect with those parts of me. I believe my body was calling for me to soften - to become more kind and gentle with myself, and to tune into myself on a physical, emotional, and spiritual level.

I began to rebuild the foundations of my mind-body connection, firstly by agreeing to listen to my body. Meditation and mindful body awareness became part of my daily practice. I began tuning in to my body and asking how it felt and what it needed. To discover just how much rest and recovery my body was requesting was confronting. It was hard for me to simply sit just for a few minutes without trying to find something productive to do, but I'm glad I stuck with it. Simply sitting and being with myself was the uncomfortable place where I began to see and know myself more fully. I was willing and curious, and even when I thought I couldn't go on growing like I was any longer, something inside of me knew that I could. Once I had made my decision to explore and express myself in a new way, there was no turning back, even when I wanted to. As soon as I would look in the direction of old comforts and habits, my body would contract and show me a clear 'No!'

To describe my journey is challenging because, like life itself, it was dynamic. There was no linear path. There were surges of growth, followed by long pauses of integration, huge a-ha moments, and lengthy periods of confusion. I spent a lot of time feeling like I was getting nowhere. The entire time though, I allowed myself to follow the thread of possibility, letting each clue lead to the next, and over time I began to understand my rhythm, my body, my nature, and what I needed to nourish my whole self. I learned the art of slowing down, and practising self-compassion. I began embracing *all* of myself, particularly the softer, slower, and simpler feminine aspects that I had suppressed for such a long time. I began cultivating a lifestyle and working with women in a way that was completely unique to me.

What I discovered was how I felt broken in more ways than I had realised.

What I learned was that the solutions and the answers that I was seeking externally had been within me all along.

What I was gifted with was a new relationship with myself, where I could sense my wholeness.

And this became the gift that I wanted to share with other women.

I began working with women in a completely new way as a physiotherapist.

When I first started working as a pelvic floor physiotherapist, I used the clinical approach that we are taught at university, one that is very much reinforced by our Western medical model. I would conduct an assessment, determine a diagnosis, and then provide a treatment plan based on the client/patient's 'problem list'. While there were many aspects of the typical Western approach to women's pelvic health that I never invited into my practice (such as offering clients solutions that meant they had to stop doing activities that they loved, and short appointment times that didn't give clients fair opportunity to ask questions and share their story) I had little awareness of the more subtle emotional and energetic body. It wasn't long before this therapeutic style didn't feel right. I knew that there was a level of embodiment that was required for women to begin to feel whole in their body that wasn't being accessed with this clinical approach. An integrated approach where science met soul needed to evolve.

The women I was working with were seeking a deeper level of healing. They were sharing that even though things looked and felt good physically, they could sense that something was off. They could sense that there was something more going on. That 'more' was the opportunity to heal beyond the physical level, and to include an emotional and energetic kind of healing. What these woman required wasn't yet another list of all the things wrong with her body and how to fix them, what they needed was an opportunity to sense their wholeness. Let me share with you one particular woman's story that was a pivotal moment in my career.

Leah (not her real name) came to me wanting to run again without pelvic symptoms. She had been working with a clinical Pilates physiotherapist after having her third baby. Pilates and physiotherapy had helped to a certain degree, but she hadn't yet been able to run again without feeling a heaviness in her pelvis. I worked with Leah, helping her to relax and soften her pelvic floor and gave her some tips on how to run with more ease. They worked, but they didn't resolve her underlying problem. One day, with tears in her eyes, Leah said to me, "Running feels good, and I get that there is nothing wrong physically, but something just doesn't feel right." I invited Leah to try one of my 3-hour Integrated Pelvic Health sessions, which she agreed to. During that session, Leah's body revealed to her the birth trauma she had experienced, how little time she had had between pregnancies and birth, and how much she was giving of herself emotionally, physically, and energetically, as well as guilt and shame that she felt around many aspects of mothering. By being present with her body, Leah was able to understand many of the emotions that were living inside of her that she was unaware of, and hadn't yet expressed. After our three hours together, she described feeling a new sense of peace and calm within her body, the peace and calm that she had been seeking, but hadn't yet found with a clinical approach. Had we continued looking at her case from a purely physical perspective, I'm not sure that this awareness would have been possible for Leah.

Over time I shifted my therapeutic approach towards a more holistic and integrative model of care that included time and space for each woman to share her story, to explore her body through movement and meditation, for her to learn what her body was showing her, and to allow her to determine her pathway towards healing through simply experiencing her body. I allowed myself to engage my intuitive wisdom, and welcomed women to do the same for themselves. Rather than me being the expert, I acknowledged that each woman is the expert in her own body, and my therapeutic approach changed to reflect that. Whilst I still use all of the therapeutic treatments that I have learned as a pelvic floor physiotherapist, how I approach my sessions is completely different.

My personal approach to women's wellness and pelvic health therapy is rooted in an understanding that there is more to us than just our physical body and that our emotional, energetic, and spiritual health have an impact on our overall wellbeing and our pelvic health and wellness. I respect the multi-layered and dynamic nature of female wellness and offer a deep acknowledgment of the emotional pain that women can carry and hold in their bodies collectively and individually. I appreciate that the pathway towards healing requires awareness and expression of this pain, and that safe spaces are required for women to explore and express their physical, emotional, and spiritual body. Sometimes, simply acknowledging, understanding, and expressing what her body is feeling, is all that is required for her to feel nourished and whole. There is power in the simplicity of being with 'what is', without trying to fix or change anything. Whatever is present for us holds purpose – it is our body's way of communicating.

Changing how I worked to become more creative and less confined by the parameters of traditional physiotherapy was challenging. I was met with an internal dialogue that made me feel trapped. I wondered what other physiotherapists would think of me, I was concerned that clients would think I was crazy, and putting myself out there on my website and in social media sharing my new vision and approach to working with women was uncomfortable. I was concerned about what people would be saying or thinking about me, but I kept myself in check by holding strong to my vision, and knowing that as long as I was maintaining full personal integrity it didn't matter what anyone else thought. I knew what women wanted and needed was very different from the old frameworks I had been using, and that moving beyond that and trusting my intuition meant I had to choose a new mindset. Changing how I approached my clinical work not only made me a better, more holistic practitioner, but my new approach also helped me cultivate deeper connections with my clients and more open and honest conversations with women, which nourished me. I was able to honour my respect for scientific evidence-based practice, while embracing the more spiritual and soulful components of myself that are essential to my own wellbeing.

I've met many women who have this same desire to bring more creativity to their work and step out of current constructs that make them feel unsatisfied and unable to reach their full potential in the work. As we connect back to our body and our nature, we feel more empowered to bring new forms of expression to our work and to our world. One of the gifts that we have living in this era is that, more and more, we can bring new ideas to life. We can break free of using the old methods that no longer serve. Creating your own path is not an easy or comfortable process, particularly in the beginning, but over time, as we find our rhythm and get to understand our creative process, and as we start to see the full spectrum of how life feels when we are expressing all parts of ourselves, there is no other way that we would have it.

I now feel so much more connected to myself, more grounded in my life, more curious, and more creative. I feel more moments of joy, and I have become more present in my life. I feel capable of being with my feelings, my emotions, and myself. I criticise myself much less often, and when I do step back into old patterns, I can redirect my mind with more ease. I am creating a life that I love, without being attached to what it looks like.

Before I tuned into my body's rhythm, I had such difficulty being present in the moment and in my body. I was always striving for more and had this constant feeling of never being quite good enough. I was off kilter. I was always doing, and never being.

Through the practices that I share in this book, I have connected more to my inherent nature and created a sense of ease in my body and in my life. I have come to realise that even though determination, dedication and self-discipline are a part of my nature, there is also calm, peace, and spaciousness available to me.

In breaking down many of my old mindsets, patterns, and beliefs, and in learning to soften, I have a completely different outlook on life. Now when I need to practice discipline, dedication and determination, I can do so with a new awareness of my whole self and I can now embrace these qualities in ways that serve me, rather than feeling exhausted and anxious. In discovering my wholeness I have been able to create a life that feels more like *me*.

I feel *whole in my skin, at home in my body, and centred in my life.*

And that is what I wish for you as well.

2

BECOMING BODY CONSCIOUS

BECOMING BODY CONSCIOUS

Many would associate being *body conscious* with feeling insecure in their body and self-conscious about how it looks or feels and what others may think about it, but my definition is different. To me, being body conscious is having a deep awareness of your body beyond how it looks, how it may be perceived, or what it can do physically/functionally. Being body conscious is *a way of being that deeply values and appreciates our body's innate intelligence to support and protect us, its wisdom that guides us from a place of truth, and being consciously aware that our body is the vessel through which we get to experience life and our wholeness.* Just as the Earth supports life, our body supports our being. Who we are goes well beyond our physical body, but it is our physical body that supports our emotional, physical and spiritual journey here in this lifetime.

This section is designed to help you to become curious about your relationship with your body, and invite you to develop a more connected relationship with your body, and your whole being.

LOVING YOUR WHOLE BODY

Loving your body is an ongoing practice. Like any relationship, your relationship with yourself and your body requires nurturing, focused energy and effort. Loving your body isn't just about being able to look in the mirror and love what you *see*, nor is it only about celebrating what your body is capable of *doing*. Whole-body love is about appreciating that your body is something that you are *living inside of,* that you get to *nurture, rest with,* and *create alongside of,* while *honouring its rhythms* and trusting its *innate wisdom.* Experiencing full body love requires us to create a relationship with our body that celebrates that it is through our physical body that we get to experience and explore life in all of its depth and vastness, and express ourselves in all of our fullness.

Your body is like your soul mate. It has always been here for you to *live* in, to *be* in, to *rely on*, and to *trust*. Your body carries and holds you through your lifetime, acting in your best interest always, even when it doesn't feel that way. By using its biological intelligence to create balance and ease, your body shows you what is good and nourishing for you. If we can sense our body for the gift that it is, rather than believing all of the things that society would tell us it is not, we realise that the physical appearance and capability of our body are just two components of our body's expression.

In this section, will we begin diving deeper into experiencing the full scope of loving your entire body as it is right now.

BODY REFLECTION JOURNAL PROMPTS AND REFLECTIVE QUESTIONS

Answer these questions honestly, without censoring yourself or thinking about what you "should" say:

- What does my body mean to me?
- My body represents...
- How do I feel in my body?
- How would I like to feel in my body? When was the last time I felt like that? What would help me to feel like that right now?
- What does 'mind-body connection' mean to me?
- My mind-body connection feels strong when...
- What does full self-expression mean to me?
- I express myself by...
- What does it feel like to feel nourished?

- I know when I am not nourishing my body and my being, because...
- I wrong my body by...
- I celebrate my body by...
- Tuning into my body's energy feels like...
- Being in my body feels easy for me when...
- I nourish my body by...
- I nourish my mind-body connection by...
- What does energetic nourishment mean to me?
- When I allow myself to move in my own rhythm I feel...

BODY CONSCIOUS LIVING

How you relate to yourself directly impacts how you relate to others. *It's all connected.* When you are disconnected from your body, you are disconnected from yourself. When you are disconnected from yourself, you distance yourself from others. Not necessarily physically, but emotionally and spiritually too. We remain disconnected from our bodies because we are afraid to feel vulnerable and uncomfortable. Instead of leaning into vulnerability, we may tense up and shut down in an attempt to control our experience. Rather than opening ourselves to our natural rhythm and letting our experiences shape us, we try to mould ourselves to what we believe others want or need us to be, trying to keep up with the demands of the outside world rather than navigating our own life using our inner compass.

When we deny ourselves the right to simply be who we truly are, we disconnect from our self, our body, other people, and our world.

When we don't believe that who we are at the core of our being is enough, we continually dishonour ourselves. We are constantly on guard, defending ourselves from a world that we believe is against us, when the real culprit is our unrelenting inner critic. Acknowledging and welcoming all parts of our self helps us to turn the volume down on our inner critic. *What pieces of yourself do you feel are not welcoming?* I was fighting my body and my need for rest, the cyclical nature of my body, my creativity, my desires, my body's wisdom, my intuition, and the parts of my physical body that I disliked. By welcoming these parts of myself through *Body Conscious* living I began to relate differently to my body, myself, my world, and to others.

The Body Conscious woman is one who lives in tune with her body's rhythms. She understands her natural cyclical state, and that moving in tune with her unique rhythm creates peace and clarity in her word. The Body Conscious woman lives in deep connection and communication with her body. She knows her body's language and is aware that living her truth feels expansive, open, peaceful, loving, and free. She senses her body's energy contracting or shrinking when she moves away from her truth and uses this guidance to find her footing again. The Body Conscious woman celebrates the gifts that come with being a woman and the wisdom that her body holds by letting her body lead and guide her. She responds to her body's needs, rather than suppressing them. She intuits her ways to optimal health, finding energetic nourishment moment by moment.

Through simple yet powerful practices, like the ones offered in this book, we offer ourselves deep connection to our body. As we become present with our body we allow ourselves to feel, and get to know, our body's language. *Whole-body love emerges and a deep trust in your body's guidance develops. This is when Body Conscious living takes place.*

OUR PAIN

It's hard to articulate the interconnected intricacies of our pain because it usually goes far beyond our physical body. The pain of deep *shame* is based on a belief that we are *broken, wrong, and not good enough* and it shows up in many ways: the mind consuming lack of self-acceptance and the endless attempts to find a way to fix ourselves, our fear around *feeling and expressing our emotions* because we believe they are unwelcome, our unwillingness to *share our truth* because we think that no one can handle it, the way that we *keep ourselves from shining too brightly*. After all there is shame in that too...

Women's pain is deep and complex.

Loving and accepting ourselves just as we are and simply being *at home* in our body are feelings/sensations that remain elusive to many women. The constant and consuming 'burden' of being a woman beats the drum of desires to be something other than we are. We feel like we need to fix ourselves in some way.

Thinner.

More toned.

Less curvaceous.

More curvaceous.

Feeling inconvenienced by our menstrual cycle.

Feeling ashamed of the natural processes of the female body.

Fighting signs of aging.

Not enjoying the pleasure of sex and intimacy, because we are worried about how we are 'performing' or concerned about how we might look.

The list goes on and on...

Our modern world and Western culture have caused us to dis-connect from our centre and abandon who we are at our core. The fierce forms of the feminine have been undernourished by the suppression of our softness, slowness, stillness, and simplicity. Not only have we tried to fit ourselves into a tight suffocating box, living in ways that uphold someone else's values, we've let go of the rituals and traditions that once served to nourish our physical, emotional and spiritual centre. When we spend our lives fighting against the natural beauty of our body, and dismissing its innate wisdom, we are left feeling undervalued, undernourished, unexpressed and overwhelmed.

From our earliest experiences of how we are introduced to our menstrual cycle, how we refer to our vulva and vagina, our experience of sex, pregnancy, birth, motherhood and beyond, there is an underlying current that reverberates the message that a woman's body is faulty in some way. Yet deep down, when we take the time to tune in, we have an inner knowing that this isn't the truth. Deep down we know that there is something *more* available to us.

Society reinforces what we have believed to be true, often through conflicting messages. How many of these messages resonate with you?

Be sexy, but not too sexy...that's slutty and scandalous.

Be confident, but not too loud or opinionated. That's irritating and embarrassing.

Ask for what you want in your work, your relationship, and in the bedroom. But don't expect to get it. That's needy and pushy!

You can do it all! Work hard and don't whinge! Successful people don't complain, they deal with it and get on with it. But you should know when to ask for help, you don't need to be a martyr!

Shhh...don't talk about that! Suppress it. Hide it. Do whatever you need to do to make it go away. Make it disappear, because we can't handle it.

Don't ask about that.

You can't ask about that!

You don't need to know how or why.

Take this pill, it will fix it.

You shouldn't have been there.

What were you doing there?

Are you sure you said no?

You're just going to have to stop doing that thing that you love so much.

Surgery is your *ONLY* option

Whilst we're there we may as well take out your uterus too.

You don't have any other options...

You can't be ready to push, we'd know if you were ready to push.

You need to push NOW!

Just be thankful you have a healthy baby, and that you are alive.

You do know that breast is best, right?

We are taught to downplay our experiences and to toughen up and get on with it. At the same time we are tormented with messages that our body is incapable and not resilient enough to cope with the natural processes of life. We have so many 'rules' to live by, and each one of them contradicts the next.

In our physical society we focus on the physical aspects of miscarriage, abortion, pregnancy, birth, and our transition into motherhood and beyond, while ignoring that these are all incredibly emotional and spiritual experiences. We are often left with heavy emotions and sensations that we push into the depths of our being, believing that our feelings are invalid or an overreaction. Besides, who has time for that when there is always so much to do?

No wonder women feel: *broken, damaged, ugly, wrong, dirty, saggy, not like a "real woman", like their bodies have failed them, inconvenient, embarrassing, chaotic and unpredictable.*

Sometimes our pain can be noisy and turbulent, but other times it's more subtle and harder to detect. Do you ever get the sensation that there is something more for you, but you don't know what? A niggle that there has to be a better way of living? Our concealed pain often tugs at our intuition, asking to be recognised. The root of our pain often stems from a learned sense of shame, but if we can gift ourselves the opportunity to unlearn our shame and answer the calls of our intuition, we can reveal more of our self and our wholeness.

FEMALE TRAUMA

When we consider female-related trauma, we often think of sexual trauma, but women's body trauma goes well beyond sexual assault and affects more than just the physical body. Women's trauma also includes birth trauma, medical trauma and surgical trauma. The causes and side effects of all of these types of trauma are both physical and emotional in nature.

Here are some examples of each:

- Birth Trauma – Feeling disempowered and uninvolved in the planning and decision making of a birth, unanticipated interventions such as unplanned C-section, vacuum assistance and/or forceps delivery, perineal tears, unhelpful or unkind comments made about the mother or baby during birth or soon after birth, baby being removed from the mother soon after birth for medical intervention.
- Medical Trauma – Feeling unsafe during pelvic exams, painful insertion of medical devices such as IUD's or catheters, feeling uninvolved in decision-making and/or uninformed around medical procedures/medications/medical interventions, language used by practitioners that causes feelings of inadequacy

or brokenness, being presented with a diagnosis in an insensitive way.

- Surgical Trauma - emotional trauma and physical symptoms related to surgical interventions such as Pelvic Organ Prolapse (POP) surgery, hysterectomy, and Dilation and Curettage surgery, being told surgery is the only option, experiencing unexpected side effects from surgical intervention.

I am not disagreeing that there are circumstances in which medical intervention is necessary. The concern is that women feel ignored, ill-informed or uninvolved in decision making around such interventions. In addition, the emotional and physical impacts are often ignored, which gives women little opportunity to seek appropriate support.

In the Western medical model, we value the scientific, evidence-based approach, which clearly has value. However, in this model of care, there is little room for a truly holistic approach that allows for women to use their intuitive knowledge and their creative wisdom to inform their healthcare choices. Valuing scientific and evidence-based practices alone means that we may miss huge opportunities that exist to simply connect to the profound wisdom we carry in our body. I believe there is room for both, and that a balanced approach is more helpful. A blend of evidence-based medicine and intuitive energetic medicine is what creates a truly holistic approach, helping to support the entire being, rather than the physical body alone.

We are very aware of the under-reporting of sexual assault and other forms of mental and physical abuse of women. We know that science is only just starting to study many of the concerns related to the female body, and that up until only recently we have seen women's bodies as too unreliable and too unpredictable to even begin to explore from a scientific standpoint because we just won't understand the data – women's bodies don't fit the scientific method of having a controlled environment. We know that when it comes to women's bodies the 'fix' that is often offered is to simply mask the symptoms with medication, because understanding the actual cause is too complex.

We know that it's a socially accepted norm that most women have a challenging relationship with their body, rooted in a sense of it not being good enough. We know how much we suppress our raw emotions because we are taught that they are unwelcome and we believe that *we* can't handle them, let alone others. For so long we have felt unseen and unheard and we've learned to shut down, stop speaking and stop expecting anything better.

It's time that we listen to our bodies, and demand that others start listening to us. We need to value our own intuitive understanding, because it is clear that in a world that values the physical and denies the intuitive, women are not receiving the standard of care that we deserve.

BODY DYSMORPHIC DISORDER

When I think about Body Dysmorphic Disorder (BDD), what immediately comes to mind is young women who have bulimia, anorexia, an eating disorder of some kind, or a compulsion for over exercising. In reality though, I believe that there is a far more common kind of BDD that women experience that we as a society accept as 'normal'.

In my teen years I experienced what it is like to have Bulimia. As a young, fit and healthy woman, it would have been easy for any outsider to see that I was experiencing body dysmorphia. What I imagined my body to look like and how it actually looked were two different things. I still don't entirely understand my experience with disordered eating, but I do know that it was very much an attempt to control how I looked. It's not an uncommon experience for young women who have been dancers, performers and gymnasts, but it doesn't matter how common it is - it's never right.

Our preoccupation with the physical appearance of our body is profound, and I believe in many ways we have come to normalise body dysmorphia. Most women can tell you that they've tried diets and rigid exercise routines, many can say they've tried pills, and perhaps even more than we would expect can admit that they've had cosmetic surgery of some description. We all know that the way women's bodies are portrayed in the media is not a true reflection of what women actually look like. We know about the airbrushing, the photo shopping, and the filters that are used. We understand that very few women are hand-picked and deemed 'good enough' to even showcase particular brands. We get it! (Even though we are sick of accepting it). What I think we understand less is the real and prevalent impact this has on women outside of the more extreme examples of eating disorders.

How many women do you know that look back at old photographs of themselves and say, "I used to think I was so fat back then, now I see clearly that I wasn't!"? Unless at some point along her path, a woman has practiced being at peace with her body, this kind of self-criticism will continue in some way. Maybe her focus will shift, but her distorted body image will continue. How much pleasure and joy do we strip from ourselves, hiding pieces of who we are that we deem not good enough? If we really sit with that and consider how much of our lives we let be consumed by trying to fix parts of ourselves that aren't even broken, we begin to sense how important it is that we begin to reclaim our relationship with our bodies.

There are far more examples of the existence of body dysmorphia amongst women, but the topics are deemed too taboo that we don't even recognise them as a problem. Let's take the vulva, for example. A woman's vulva rarely looks like the images displayed not only in porn but also in medical texts and health information resources. We are getting better as a society at recognising that women that work within the sex/porn industry are often expected to have cosmetic surgery to alter the appearance of their vulva through labiaplasty surgery, but rather than embracing what is normal, labiaplasty surgery rates continue to rise. According to the American Society of Aesthetic Plastic Surgery Statistics (2017), labiaplasty is up 217.2% from 2012 to 2017.

We are also beginning to recognise from a scientific health care perspective that we have probably been *over-diagnosing prolapse* from a clinical measurement scale because we now have studies to show that what was being determined as a grade one (1) prolapse is actually *normal movement of the vaginal walls.* (Buchsbaum et el., 2006; Dietz et el., 2016; Harmanli, 2014) Yes, your vaginal walls are meant to have movement! What I see increasingly in my clinic, are women who believe that their vaginal wall movement is excessive/wrong/not normal, and that they have a prolapse, even though upon assessment they have what is clinically determined as normal vaginal wall movement. Sometimes it's because someone has diagnosed them with having a prolapse, and sometimes it's because they simply didn't have an understanding that the vaginal walls are meant to move – perhaps because our society has an unrealistic view of what vaginas are meant to look and feel like, stemming from the pornographic obsession with women having 'tight' vaginas.

BEYOND THE BODY

As human beings, we tend to see our world in a very physical way because we can make sense of it. What exists beyond the physical can seem intangible, unexplainable, and esoteric. Sometimes when we are unable to explain something or witness it in its physical form we negate its realness. When we have scientific evidence to explain something we feel confident in its truth and it's the subtler energetic and spiritual aspects of life that can be hard to wrap our head around, and when something is difficult to understand we question its value and its truth. This can happen even though at a deeper level we understand what we can't quite describe with words.

When we have physical complaints and we look at them from a purely physical perspective, we can miss the more subtle energetic, emotional, and spiritual contributors to the problem. With this narrow perspective, we offer ourselves a limited scope of healing potential and possibility. We become frustrated, feeling like no one is hearing or understanding us, and no one can help us find a progressive pathway.

The universal experience of pain can help us to understand why it's often important that we go beyond the physical body to heal our physical symptoms. The concepts that follow are also useful for women who may not have a physical complaint but would like to experience life with more ease. Gaining clarity on the interconnectedness of our mind, body, and spirit can demonstrate why an integrated approach to our wellness is helpful and can have a profound impact.

What we know from science is that 100% of the time physical pain is created by our brain. Pain is a protective mechanism that serves to warn us of danger and keep us safe. When pain receptors in our body detect an episode of acute injury, they send messages to different parts of our body, including our brain, where this information is deciphered using the current information, along with stored memory. Our brain then determines how much of a threat we are under and decides on an appropriate response. Your brain then stores this episode as a memory to make sure that the next time we experience a similar situation we can act accordingly (Butler and Moseley, 2013).

What we also know from science is that *pain is not an accurate measure of tissue health*. Sometimes we can experience very real and persistent pain in the absence of ongoing tissue damage, often known as chronic pain or persistent pain. In the instance of chronic pain, the signal can become too persistent, giving us unnecessary warning signs. Another amazing thing about pain is that it can occur in the absence of *any* physical stimuli. Thoughts and places can activate the warning signals, and your brain can create a very real pain sensation in response. This is sometimes referred to as psychosomatic pain, and has until recently been dismissed as "all in your head". Only recently have practitioners begun to understand that this type of pain is no less real to the person experiencing it. Chronic pain is complex and is *less about* the structural body and tissues, and *more about the neurobiological system*. In other words, *chronic pain is less about our physical body and more about our mind-body connection*. Chronic pain has more to do with our biological, social, emotional, environmental, and cultural experiences associated with pain over time. Stress and anxiety are two well-known contributors to this type of pain. Research shows that a physical approach alone towards managing, improving, and treating chronic pain is limited. In order to best manage chronic pain we need to *retrain the brain*. We need to understand the deeper thoughts, emotions and beliefs that co-create the experience of pain, along with the environmental stimuli. (Butler and Mosely, 2013)

Using pain as an example, we can see that our state of well-being goes far beyond our physical experience. A complex interplay exists between our mind, our body, our environment, and our experience. Although I've used pain as an example, I don't believe this complex interplay pertains to our experience of pain alone, but our experiences with our mind and body as a whole. Just as treating chronic pain requires a neural rewiring that considers the complexities of our mind-body relationship and our experiences, a wide scope approach is required for all kinds of women's pain – physical, emotional and spiritual. From unsuccessful attempts to maintain a "healthy weight", to treating pelvic organ prolapse, to creating a lifestyle that feels aligned, rewarding and fulfilling, a whole-body integrated approach to wellbeing is what women are seeking and what we need.

TAKING PERSONAL RESPONSIBILITY

It wouldn't be fair to blame our collective lack of body love and body acceptance on one specific factor alone. The media, the health and fitness industry, social constructs and expectations of what a woman's body should look like and how it should function and learned behaviours that come from a long lineage of women who also lacked body acceptance, are all complex factors in our collective disembodiment. Placing blame, however, is an ineffective strategy to try to overcome the lack of self-worth and body appreciation that we experience internally. *The process and practice of learning self-love, self-appreciation, and self-acceptance has to start from within.* It begins and ends with you. Placing blame takes away from our autonomy and our personal responsibility. This same autonomy and responsibility give us the opportunities to create growth and change, both on a personal and collective level.

To separate ourselves from the exploitation and social expectations of women and their bodies, we need to journey inward and build a strong and healthy relationship with our whole selves. Placing the blame onto others, and trying to make it someone else's responsibility won't work. We need to take responsibility for what we are willing to create and accept for ourselves.

Before I continue, I want to make something very clear. There are situations in life where we are unable to keep ourselves safe. There are times when another person or people take advantage of us and we experience trauma through NO fault of our own. Taking personal responsibility is not about blaming ourselves for traumatic experiences, and knowing this important difference is key. In the instance of trauma, we must acknowledge that the trauma affects different systems of functioning in the brain, and has an impact physically, emotionally, and cognitively. Self-empowerment and choice become apparent when the trauma is first acknowledged, and ownership is taken over navigating the pathway forward with appropriate support networks (professional and personal) in place.

With that understanding of the key difference between self-blame versus personal ownership of experience that does not relate to trauma, it's important to realise that you get to choose the life that you live. Your world, as you know it, exists within the mind and the body that you live in. You are both the narrator of your story and the character you play. You get to choose how you feel and how you respond to life. You are in control of the inner workings of your world. You get to decide how life is working *against you*, or how life is working *for you*. We don't get to control the actions of others, and we don't get to control everything that happens in life but the moment we start blaming someone or something else for how we feel is the moment that we put ourselves under the illusion that that person/thing/event has control over us. The moment we blame someone else for how we feel, we hand over our personal power. We have a choice, we can choose to fall victim to our circumstances or someone else's actions or we can choose to win back the only real control we have in our life, which is to create the world in which we live – the world that exists within our own mind and body.

LISTEN INWARD

Depending on your relationship with your body, you may not pay much attention to it unless it's telling you that there is something wrong. This is like only paying attention to your child when they are requesting something, reacting to their articulated needs alone, rather than nurturing a loving and curious relationship that invites conversation and welcomes a depth of knowledge and understanding by listening with keen interest. The difference between the two relationships and the wellbeing of that child would be significant, and we all know what child we would rather be. Only reacting to pain, discomfort, and illness is a very different way of relating to your body as opposed to nurturing a curious relationship that is connected, open, and aware. How well we feel in our body will depend on the relationship that we create with it. How well we expect to feel in our body depends on what we believe is possible and what we expect wellness to feel like. Grab a notebook and brainstorm some responses to these questions:

What does optimal wellness feel like to me?

Is it simply a lack of disease and pain?

Could I be expecting more?

Optimal wellness comes from a sense of wholeness. A sense of wholeness is developed when we can embrace all parts of our being, when we permit ourselves to fully express our self, knowing that we are capable of feeling uncomfortable, and when we welcome all parts of our self, rather than becoming self-critical, we are able to simply observe our experience with self-compassion. Optimal wellness is a state of calm and peace, and an understanding that even though challenging moments and emotions will arise, we have the strength and ability to move through them by feeling them, expressing them, and simply seeing the experience for what it is, rather than becoming so attached to it that it begins to define us and/or our experience of life.

To experience an optimal state of wellbeing, we need to create a relationship that goes beyond simply responding to our body's warning signals and facilitate a more open conversation with our body. We need to go beyond the body and bring our attention to our thoughts, beliefs, and emotions and become aware of how we react or respond to them. We need to sense the interconnectedness of all things beyond the physical realm. In understanding and appreciating our physical, energetic, emotional, and spiritual body, we gift ourselves more opportunity to sense our wholeness.

PRACTICING BODY PRESENCE

Practicing body presence doesn't mean that you will always feel good in your body but part of practicing body presence is knowing that feeling good NOW is readily available to you. It kind of depends on what you define as 'good'. Good can mean that you feel energetic, alive, and radiant. Feeling 'good' can also mean that you are simply capable of accepting how you feel no matter how that is. You can feel tired and accept that. You can feel confused and unsure and accept that. When you can accept how you feel, it no longer has a hold on you – and that's what body presence and feeling good is about. It's about acceptance. Acceptance is a huge part of Body Conscious living because allowing yourself to accept how you feel also allows you to nourish your body in the way it desires.

BREAKING THE MOULD AND STOPPING THE CYCLE

As we bring more awareness to our centre, we connect more to our truth. As we connect more to our truth we sense how we can express ourselves more fully and how we would like to feel in our life. When we know who we are at our core, and what creates a life that feels good to us, we begin to move from a place of knowing, become more aligned with our centre and be more our self. We realise where in our lives we have conformed to societal constructs and begin the challenging and uncomfortable process of breaking free from moulds and stepping outside of the boxes we have confined ourselves to. This revealing of self is unique to each of us.

The following practices and prompts are designed to help you to connect to your centre, and sense where you may like to create new ways of being. This is not a step-by-step guide. Use what resonates and trust your inner knowing - it will be your best guide.

KNOW HOW YOU REALLY WANT TO
FEEL IN YOUR BODY

Knowing how you want to feel in your body and how to ignite that feeling helps us to bring us closer to living our truth. Often we are chasing a feeling by taking actions that don't actually get us closer to experiencing how we really want to feel. For example, we try diet after diet in an attempt to lose weight, believing that once we lose it we will feel good. Meanwhile we despise the diet itself as well as how we feel in our body. No quicker than we lose the weight, we put it on again. The diet is unenjoyable and unsustainable, and we don't end up experiencing the sensation of feeling good in our body, which was the whole purpose of the diet. This is because are trying to ignite a sense of self-worth by focusing on how badly we feel at our current weight. *We continue to hold onto the physical and energetic weight of not believing in our self-worth.*

Although a good understanding of nutrition, choosing real foods, and movement are requirements for maintaining a healthy weight, when we continue to hold onto the energetic weight of not feeling whole and comfortable in our skin we continue to feel heavy and our body reflects that. Connecting to the sensations of how we want to *feel in our body* and allowing them to gain momentum is a far more helpful and satisfying experience than trying to commit to yet another diet and exercise regime that actually makes you feel like you are being punished.

Another common example that I see in my practice is postnatal women who believe what they want is to look and feel the same way they did prior to pregnancy. Generally what these women really want to feel is *strong, capable, and at peace in their body.* The impatience of wanting to be somewhere we are not, and trying to control our experience in an attempt to feel something that we don't, creates a sensation that our *body is failing us.* This makes us think that how we want to feel is out of reach and impossible. Instead, if we were to sense our strength and meet ourselves where we are in a way that feels connected, we would ignite the sensations of being strong and capable of being able to move through this transition phase with ease. We would be able to feel the strength and capability we are seeking.

The more we focus more on how we *don't want to feel*, and what we need to fix, the more we give meaning and momentum to the 'problem' that we think needs fixing. Knowing how you want to feel and igniting more of that energy and emotion helps manifest more of that energy and emotion in your life.

This next practice may help you:

- Become aware of your thought patterns, and the energy that is attached to them
- Become aware of where in your body/life you are thinking something needs to be fixed
- Become aware of where you focus on the problem, giving it more momentum
- Become clear about how you *do* want to *feel*
- Know what ignites that feeling within you
- Practice igniting and staying in that energy more often

Knowing what feels expansive, open, and true in your body is a great way to connect to your truth and know how you want to feel. The Deep Core Connection Practice (p. 273 - 277) helps you connect to your deep core so that you can sense how your body responds to different thoughts, feelings, and actions. Aligned thoughts, feelings and actions create openness within. Your breath will feel calm, your muscles will feel relaxed, and your energy will feel expansive. When thoughts, feelings, and actions cause your energy to contract, your muscles to become tense, and cause your breathing to become fast or restricted, this is your body showing you that these thoughts/feelings/actions are not aligned with your centre or your truth. Tuning into your body's sensations can help you to know when you are moving from a place of truth and when you may need to adjust your course.

Practicing body presence and being where you are, as is, *is the practice*. Accepting where we are, and allowing ourselves to feel good in our body as it is in this moment allows us to access the peace and joy that we are seeking. When we continue to push our body to be other than it is, we are hoping that when we are something other than what we are, we will feel good. We are practicing not being satisfied with our body as it is now. The neurological pattern that continues to be reinforced is "I am not good enough" and "I need to be different to feel good".

When we practice body presence by bringing awareness to ourselves and our body as it is in this moment, we can relax and expand into the moment that we are experiencing now through the body that we are living in *now*. Feelings of ease are evoked and we begin to practice how it feels to be content, joyful, and at peace in our body.

This doesn't mean that we don't sleep well, eat poorly, avoid exercise, and simply say, "When I practice feeling present in my body, I feel well.' Body Conscious living makes it easy for us to make choices that are nourishing for our body and good for our well-being. When we practice body presence we move for energetic nourishment, not punishment, we enjoy nurturing our being and our body, rather than feeling that maintaining our health and wellbeing is a burden.

Reflect on the following questions:

- How would I like to feel in my body and in my life?
- Where in my life do I already feel that?
- What qualities and parts of myself am I bringing to these "feel good" parts of my life that I can invite to the parts of my life that don't feel so good? (i.e. - my strength, positivity, determination)

TRANSITION AND CHANGE ARE NATURAL, NORMAL, AND HEALTHY

We are obsessed with fighting our natural progression of aging. We have created and subscribed to a dialogue that says that as you age you decrease in your value, become less capable of feeling good in your body and that aging is ugly. Hide it at all costs! These stories stop us from embracing our transitions across our life cycle.

I hear 40-year-old women talking about 20-year-old women, and how beautiful, fit and thin they are, but did these 40-year-old women think that of themselves when they were 20? Maybe now in hindsight these women can see their own beauty at 20 years of age, but often they had the same body image concerns 20 years ago that they do now. I hear 60-year-old women say to 40-year-old women, "What I would give to be able to move my body like you can!" but when that 60-year-old woman was 40 years of age, did she feel the joy and freedom of being in her body? Or was she fixated on how her 'post-baby body' didn't move with the same ease and strength that it once did? You get my point.

We have a choice. Accept our body as it is now, enjoy it, and give ourselves the chance to love it or keep trying to be back *there*, 5, 10, or 15 years ago, when we also hated our body.

FIND THE FEELING PRACTICE

- Find a comfortable position, close your eyes and connect to your breath.
- Sense how you currently feel in your body.
- Consider how you would like to feel in your body right now.
- Recall the last time you felt like this in your body and let that feeling wash over you. Imagine how this sensation would smell, taste, and feel in your body.
- Once you have connected to the feeling ask your body, "How can I ignite this feeling in my life today?"
- Use your body's response to guide your actions.

SOFTEN

One of the most challenging things about connecting to and living from your centre is learning to soften. Softening begins with being vulnerable and honest with yourself about how you really feel. This can feel uneasy, particularly when we believe that we are not capable of processing big emotions and that our emotions are wrong or unwelcome. For some, dropping into the body is challenging and confronting. Combining self-love, self-kindness, and self-compassion with the simple act of observing your feelings without judgement, or attaching a story to how you feel, is an incredibly powerful practice that helps us soften from within. Creating safe spaces to feel seen, heard, and witnessed in our softness is even more powerful.

CREATING SAFE SPACES FOR FEELINGS TO BE SEEN, HEARD, AND WITNESSED

The simple act of carving out space and time for your feelings to be seen, heard, and witnessed can reveal parts of yourselves that you might not even know exist. Women go through so many transitions across their lifespan and simply having a space to talk about our experience(s), to reflect, and to notice how we feel opens an incredible path that leads to our softening. When we don't have these opportunities to reflect, connect, and process these transitions, our body begins to hold onto the energetic residue. This residue can intensify over time, and morph into physical symptoms such as pelvic pain, pain with intercourse, jaw and neck pain, irritable bowel syndrome, constipation, and bloating. Some women become disinterested in sex, even though they want to be interested in sex, while others experience increasing period pain or symptomatic change/s in their menstrual cycle. When we ignore our experiences, our body finds a way to draw our attention to them.

Finding spaces where you can feel safe to be vulnerable with your emotions can seem difficult. As a society, we don't place value in creating such spaces, and so they are less prominent, but they do exist. Creating these spaces is part of my work, and part of the reason for this book is to call more women to create these spaces for themselves. The challenge in creating these opportunities for ourselves is that sometimes when we talk to our loved ones, in their efforts to support us, they often want to 'fix' things by giving advice, or by trying to show us how to redirect our emotions rather than feeling them. The very purpose of these spaces, though, is to help you to soften into yourself so that you can see that you are not broken and that you have the capability, resilience, and strength to be present with, and move through, your emotions.

Being present with the sensations we feel and expressing emotions helps our body to process rather than hold onto them physically and energetically. Finding a coach, a therapist, or a practitioner who is practiced in witnessing and listening without always offering a solution or a fix is important. This doesn't mean that they won't be able to help you. It simply means that you become more autonomous in your own care and healing.

TRUST YOUR INTUITION

Throughout this book, there are practices that create opportunities for you to connect with your body's wisdom and your inner knowing. As you engage with these practices, ideas or thoughts will likely arise that don't seem to make logical sense. Your mind may question your judgement and offer you all of the reasons that your intuition/guidance/insight cannot be right or true. Our mind plays an important role in critical thinking and offering discernment. We don't need to cast judgement over our thoughts or try to stop them from being there; rather we simply ask our critical thinking brain to take a step back. Use your discernment, but also trust your intuition. It can be difficult to know the difference between your mind and your intuition, and being comfortable with trusting your intuition takes practice.

Here are some ways that I decipher whether I am getting caught up in my mind, or if I am connected to my intuition. Try them for yourself and see what feels good.

- Using the Deep Core Connection Practice (p. 273 - 277) or any of the Womb Energy Connection Practices (p. 279- 281) to help tune into your body's energy and ask your body for guidance. Trust that whatever guidance is received in that moment is your intuition/your body's knowing/ your body's wisdom. If you have two opposing thoughts/opinions/options, sense how your core energy responds to each thought. Generally one thought will feel more expansive, open, and peaceful in your core; whilst the other may feel contracted, closed, and tense. The thought/option that feels more expansive is what your intuition is guiding you towards.

- A thought/idea that seems to come from nowhere, with more a sense of it being right and less an attachment to the outcome and feels like 'I just know, but I have no idea why!' is more likely to be your intuition.

- A thought that seems more repetitive and 'hooks' you into creating a story around the likely outcome of a particular action, that snowballs into other thoughts concerning *the how* is more likely to be your Ego trying to crush your intuition.

As you learn to trust your intuitive guidance, play with something small first. Experiment with something that feels safe and easy rather than a make or break decision. I sold our family home and moved interstate off a hunch. I use my intuition to create all of my therapeutic offerings and guide business decisions. However, this all comes off the back of practicing using my body's guidance with less critical life decisions like 'How will I move my body today?', or 'What would feel good to enjoy as a family activity today?'. Over time this progressed to my body guiding my days – where, for example, I would structure my day based on my body's guidance rather than the clock. Much later this progressed to making bigger life decisions based on intuitive guidance.

If understanding your body's language feels very new to you, the following practice may help you tap into your intuition:

- Find a quiet place to relax, either sitting or lying, and drop into your body by focusing on your breath.
- Begin making statements that you KNOW to be true. For example, "I love my dog", "I hate Liquorish," or "Coffee is my favourite drink."
- Pay close attention to how your body feels when you make these statements. Does any tension arise? Do you feel comfortable? You may smile, or feel pleasant sensations.
- Take a break for a few minutes and go do something else.
- Return to your quiet place and drop into your body again.
- This time, reverse the statements so that you KNOW they are false. "I hate my dog!" or "Liquorish is delicious!"
- Notice how your body responds, paying close attention to your gut. You may feel a contraction, or almost a wave of nausea.

- Practice this exercise as a way to develop your intuition and as a way to 'warm up' before accessing your intuition to make larger decisions.

STOP ASKING OTHERS ABOUT WHAT'S RIGHT FOR YOUR BODY - IT'S ALREADY TOLD YOU

Whether it's the obvious rejection of a particular medication, including the side effects of contraception that the doctor reassures you are 'normal' even though you sense that something just doesn't feel right, or the pain you're experiencing from the new exercise regime, or the bloating you feel after eating a particular food – EVERY SINGLE TIME, your body is giving you clear signals that 'this is not agreeing with you'.

In my conversations with women, I hear things like, "I've been told to use this contraception by my GP, and personally I would prefer not to be using any hormonal contraception, but she said I should, and so I am." or "You will say I should be doing my pelvic floor exercises, but I when I was doing them I was getting pelvic pain, and so I stopped". Your body is YOURS! No one knows your body the way you do. Your body knows what it needs, and it's communicating with you all the time. Trust it.

QUESTION WHAT YOU BELIEVE

Make it a practice to question what you believe to be true. I used to believe that job security was important to me. I also believed that finding work that I loved was impossible and that if I did that it would pay poorly. When I started tuning into my centre more deeply, it showed a different truth. My body knew that I could create opportunities for myself to work in ways that I loved, and that joy and freedom were more important to me than job security. When we open ourselves up and get to know who we are at the core of our being, we naturally begin to question what we believe to be true. Open yourself to the process.

When you resist taking action that would bring you closer to realising your desires, be curious about what unconscious belief is stopping you by simply asking yourself, "What is the underlying belief that is stopping me from taking the next best step?" Ultimately you get to choose what you believe.

Contemplate the following:

- How are your beliefs serving you?
- Does your mindset keep you open to opportunity? Or do your beliefs close you off from your creative potential?
- How is your mindset working for you or against you?

When you bring your awareness to limiting beliefs, you have the opportunity to choose something different for yourself. Play around with reframing your beliefs.

- What would it feel like to believe the complete opposite to what you currently believe?
- How does that feel in your body?
- Can you find a new belief that feels exciting, but also feels true?
- How would moving from this deeper truth look?

The success of mindset reprogramming is dependent on connecting with a deeper truth that resonates with us. Again, finding our deeper truth requires an exploration of what beliefs and thoughts feel contracted, tense and untrue, versus beliefs that feel relaxed, open, and expansive. Once you discover what feels true and aligned for you, you get to play in the realm of new beliefs. Each time you sense yourself reverting to old thought patterns, you can catch yourself, and redirect your thinking to affirm your new belief system. Create ways of being that confirm your new beliefs and add to your conscious and subconscious evidence that supports them. Talk out loud about your new belief systems to yourself and others. Open your imagination and play with creating new beliefs and notice how life begins to feel and look different for you.

BREAK THE RULES

Much of what holds us back from living from our centre is an illusion that we need to follow some set of unwritten rules. We conform to acting in ways that we believe are socially acceptable because we're concerned about what someone might think of us. We tell ourselves things like, "I can't quit my job, my colleagues would be so disappointed and my in-laws will think I am lazy". Firstly, we don't know what others would think unless we have asked them. Secondly, others aren't thinking about us even half the amount of time we imagine them to be. Lastly, does it matter what they think? Five years from now would you rather be in a job that isn't right for you because you think it makes your colleagues and in-laws happy? Or would you rather be in a job that is right for you that makes you happy? Ultimately this type of mindset projects blame onto others for how we are choosing to create our life. Rather than taking ownership and personal responsibility for our actions, we make excuses by blaming others for how our life is. Stepping up and claiming your creative power is taking radical personal responsibility for the life you are creating.

We are not born as unique as we are only to spend our lives trying to morph ourselves into a carbon copy that someone else created and deemed valuable. Don't you think it's more believable that we were born with our own special desires, skills, and challenges so that we can create a life that is unique to us? Our Earth is not filled with the vastness of life and such a variety of species by mistake. They all serve their purpose in helping our planet's interconnected and complex ecosystem to thrive. Imagine if all of the bird species in the world tried to be like one another, trying to morph the colours of their feathers, their mating dances, and the sound of their birdsong to be like another kind of bird species. It would be impossible and pointless. It's the same for us as human beings. When we live by our own rules, pave our own way, and create a unique life that is aligned to our own set of core values we get to live our divine purpose. This illusion that we need to follow the rules and be like someone else only keeps us small as individuals and stops us from seeing our full potential as human beings.

YOU CAN'T GET IT WRONG

Do what you've always done, feel how you've always felt. Do something differently, feel something different. Simple right? What if you couldn't get your life wrong? What if every action was in service of your personal growth and in service of everything you are here to feel, observe, and experience? We are so afraid of getting it wrong. Worrying about where this might lead, how this will end up, what someone else might think. Not doing what you want to, not living full out, is the greatest disservice we could do to ourselves, to others and to the opportunity of life. We only get one shot at living this life in this body. If we let the amplitude of that resonate through our being, we can see how ridiculous it is living your life for someone else. That's not what your life was designed for. That is not what you signed up for when you said yes to come into this reality. What you signed up for was to experience life. So, if you can't get this wrong, what is it you want to experiment with or to try differently so that you give yourself more opportunity to create the life that you want to create?

OPEN TO POSSIBILITY AND POTENTIAL

I remember when I started on my own journey; my heart and mind became open to new potential and possibility. I could see how I could create a life that felt more aligned and alive. I was excited by possibility, my husband became concerned: "Don't get your hopes up, I don't want you to get disappointed". I told him I was well practiced at failure and that being disappointed wasn't anything that I hadn't experienced before. It was worth the risk to move in the direction of my desires while believing anything is possible than to stay put in this illusionary 'safe zone' in a career that didn't light me up, in a world where others dictated when I would be at work, when I would be at home and when I was allowed to take holidays. Our fear of taking risks, failing, and the disappointment we might feel if things don't turn out how we hope can be debilitating, but we also know that without taking a risk we will continue to create much of the same. Without 'failure' we don't have the opportunities to learn and grow. When life doesn't pan out the way that we hoped we are very capable of moving through it. Alternatively, things turn out way better than we anticipated or imagined and we are left pinching ourselves at what we have been able to create.

To be honest, when I first started in my business I had a vision of creating an online million dollar business that offered me the time freedom and financial freedom that I desired. I imaged creating a successful business with loads of passive income. Back then that's what I thought I wanted. Having worked my arse off trying to do that, I realised that creating a 'passive income' was time-consuming, and that creating a successful online business was really hard work (doing it in the way that I was) and that didn't it offer the time and freedom I was craving at all. In my attempt to create an online business, my value of freedom was severely sacrificed. What I also discovered was that I wasn't prepared to create a business in a way that felt forced and full of effort. I realised that trying to follow in the footsteps of others by using their '10 Steps to Success' didn't feel like success to me. It felt exhausting. I wouldn't have discovered this if I didn't dive in and give it a go. I would have continued to work in a job that I disliked imagining that there could be a better life out there, but it wasn't for me because I didn't have what it takes. Instead, I have evolved into creating a lifestyle business that is totally *me* and aligned with my values.

We are taught not to ask for more, or to expect more. At the same time, we are taught all the ways that we need to be more which naturally leads us to seek more. The problem is that we seek 'more' in all of the wrong places because we don't even know what it is that we are looking for. In this instance, what we think we want/need to create a life that feels alive and what we actually need are totally different things. If we simply permitted ourselves to connect with our innermost desires, to believe in our personal potential and in the possibility of aligned living, and to follow our desire with the next best step, we would see our lives unfolding in ways that feel more like us and less like someone told us it should. We would create a life that feels in tune with our personal values and unique vision. We would appreciate the journey and see how life is working for us and never against us. This is what creates a life well-lived.

Living a life that you feel is expected of you is like going on a holiday, packing someone else's suitcase, and trying to explore your surroundings using some else's map and itinerary which gives directions to destinations that belong to a place on the other side of the world. You would feel lost, unsatisfied, and your holiday wouldn't feel like a holiday at all! Until maybe you decide to ditch the ill-fitting clothes, the map, and the itinerary and just make it up as you go along – now that sounds like fun!

BODY LED LIVING

Challenging ourselves to consider how we move through our world, where we are not being true to ourselves, and how we might like to create new ways of being is a lot to try and navigate. There is no linear pathway. It's more like a treasure hunt created by a three-year-old genius with a huge imagination. Multiple paths lead in many different directions, but somehow all come back to one centre. On seeking the treasure you find little clues along the way, with lots of special surprises and some hard lessons earned. Sometimes you think you're walking in one direction, then realise you actually want to be on a different path, and because there are no definite rules to follow you can redirect your path at any time. Maybe you try to escape a lesson by navigating in a different direction, but this magical treasure hunt is like a matrix that fosters great flexibility and creativity and the lesson finds you in a new way. Your hunt is like nobody else's. Your path is like no other. Where you choose to go is completely up to you!

You might like to think of this book as a companion on your path that will offer some integral pieces of understanding and practices to help you along your way. Your journey will be unique, where you choose to focus your attention and how much time you need to spend with each component is for you to decide. In creating this book I knew there was no one perfect way to organise its content because the work is so interconnected and integrative. I've created it in a way that makes sense to me, and my experience. You will read and use this book in whatever way feels right for you. I completely trust that however you decide to approach this book and the practices within will be perfect for you.

OPENING THE CONVERSATIONS ABOUT WOMEN'S BODIES

As a general population, we know very little about the female body. When we compare what is generally known about a male body to what is known about the female body, it becomes obvious how little conversation and education exists around the female body. We know men have a penis and two scrota, that when men become aroused there is an increase in blood flow that causes their penis to become erect, and that during an orgasm a man ejaculates sperm, and that is part of what is required for procreation. Compare that common knowledge to our understanding of the female anatomy and genitalia. Most women don't even know the correct terminology of their outer genitalia (which is the vulva by the way) let alone have an understanding of the female menstrual cycle. We have a hard time just saying vulva and vagina, let alone knowing the difference! To be completely honest I found it difficult when I first started teaching my girls about their vulvas using the correct terminology. It wasn't because I found it uncomfortable, but because I imagined that when they use the correct terminology others would feel awkward! I observe the internal discomfort and continue to do what feels right, which is teaching my children about their body and continue to break down the shame barriers that exist within myself and in society.

For so long we as a society have been under the illusion that women's bodies are like 'small men'. We are taught that the difference between a man and a woman's body, apart from the obvious anatomical difference of genitalia, is that we have less strength, power, and endurance. We are less able to build muscle mass, and therefore perform at a different level in sports. That's it! But we don't talk about the physiological and anatomical differences that are the obvious differences because they are too taboo, or we don't know enough about them yet.

I have seen male personal trainers who specialise in postnatal fitness say that there is no difference between the female and male pelvic floor. That might seem like I'm taking a small minority and putting a blanket description over a wider population, but it isn't unusual for male or female fitness professionals to claim that they specialise in postnatal or female specific training when the only understanding that they have of what's particularly unique about a postnatal woman is that she's probably getting less sleep than the average person and that she has a baby. Yes, this is a problem that could be better managed by the industry, but this is just one example of a problem that exists on a much larger scale.

In a health care setting, women are often told by their GP's or gynaecologist to do their pelvic floor exercises and then, if that doesn't help, surgery is their next option. There is often no recommendation to have an internal pelvic floor assessment to determine what may be the cause of the patient's concerns and therefore what options she has to help improve her overall wellbeing and little consideration for the multifaceted and ongoing impacts of that surgery or their usually very low success rate.

We have structures in place for workers compensation for injury related to the workplace, but what woman is ever going to tell her boss that her uterus prolapsed during a work incident? Particularly when we live in a culture where:

1. The woman would feel such shame around it that she would keep it a secret and maybe not even talk to her GP about it, let alone her boss;
2. The woman's body would likely be to blame, rather than the incident and;
3. Depending on what health care providers she comes across in her journey she would be told her options are either to stop work or have surgery.

On one hand, women are constantly told the pain that they feel in their body is either in their head or normal. On the other hand, we pathologise normal and healthy events like sometimes-irregular periods, pregnancy, and birth. How are women expected to know when they should seek medical assistance? How are women meant to know when their experience is normal and healthy, or when what they feel is a symptom of something that requires medical or professional support? Unless we have a good understanding of our body, and unless we can trust in our understanding of it, we can feel lost and less able to make well-informed decisions that are imperative for our overall health and wellbeing.

We need to know our body from a functional and physical health perspective. Perhaps even more importantly, we need to know our body intimately so that we are able to enjoy the full spectrum of the pleasures that life has to offer. Recall back at the start of this book where I explained how our relationship with our self and our body affects every aspect of our life. It affects our mood, our relationships, our internal motivation, our creativity, and our willingness to participate. It affects *everything*. If we don't know our own body, how can we optimise our experience of life? If we don't think that's important as a society, then why do we spend so much time and money trying to sell things we don't even need by telling us how they are going to make our life better in some way?

WHAT IS THE FEMININE?

Feminine energy is very different from masculine energy, but at the same time, they are not separate. This can be a difficult concept to wrap your head around. This is the concept of duality and polarity, which is evident everywhere in life. For me, this concept became most evident when I became more aware of the parts that existed within me that I had been suppressing. Parts of me that seemed to be opposite or contradictory to who I knew myself to be. I often felt like a walking contradiction. I am a mover. I love momentum. Movement is my medicine. When I have a creative block I go for a run, and I become inspired. At the same time, I love stillness, slowness, and simplicity. The slower I go in my life, the more I feel joy in the movement. These are contradictory and opposite natures that exist within me.

Feminine energy is often described as softer, less energetic, more creative, and more abstract whereas masculine energy is considered to be more logical and analytical. Neither is right nor wrong. They complement one another. When some people talk about being in flow, they talk about being in their feminine energy. I consider a state of flow as being able to flex between the phases where my masculine energy is more prominent and other times where I call more upon my feminine energy. I like to think of a surfer out in the ocean, sitting in the stillness waiting for the perfect wave to ride. This stillness is her calm and peaceful feminine energy but it's not separate from her masculine energy that she is using to read the waves and detect which one she will chase next. When she is riding the wave she's perhaps more in her masculine energy, moving with strength and speed, but this is not separate from her feminine state where she is feeling completely at home in her body, in the zone, and at one with nature. This is how I sense the masculine and feminine as different yet intertwined states of being. One can't thrive without the other to support it. This is where we often slip up as a collective. We have suppressed our feminine energy, thinking that the 'more is more' approach and constantly *do*ing is the path to success when, in reality, suppressing the feminine stifles creativity, creates huge amounts of stress and anxiety, and takes the joy out of life. When we talk about the rise of the feminine, we aren't hoping that feminine energy will someday dominate over masculine energy. We are hoping that we can invite and create more balance in the way we approach life.

THE FORGOTTEN FEMININE

In some self-help and spiritual realms, it would appear that the path to awakening the forgotten feminine is through becoming au fait with crystals, oracle cards, and the use of Yoni eggs. While these can be beautiful ways to connect with different aspects of our self, this is *not* what creates true feminine connection. If you think about the feminine and imagine floral floaty dresses and young children running around in beautiful white garments singing and dancing in the garden while their mother meditates and drinks herbal tea amongst the wildflowers, I'd say you're not alone! That image used to come to my mind often when I thought about the feminine. I don't believe this is an impossible vision to manifest, and that it couldn't be part of our real world, but at the same time, I don't believe this is an entirely accurate description of what real feminine expression looks like, at least not for every woman. Even for those women who do have an experience like I've described above, expressing their feminine wouldn't *always* look like this. To me, remembering the feminine, awakening the feminine, and embracing the feminine is simply allowing yourself to open to parts of you that you have perhaps suppressed or ignored over time. Certainly, it's about looking for patterns of behaviour that reflect societal values rather than our own and offering ourselves a new opportunity to live in a way that is more reflective of our true and unique nature. Awakening the feminine is more about *being more you* than anything else.

For many women this means:

- Slowing down
- Becoming more creative in how we approach our work and our life
- Paving our unique path
- Getting to know, understand and respect our body and respond to its needs by finding physical and energetic nourishment moment by moment
- Being present with our emotions, thoughts, feelings, and sensations
- Knowing and speaking our truth
- Becoming aware of societal pressure and constructs that we have followed, and
- Rewiring our mind-body pathways to create new ways of being that feel more true and aligned

There is no right way to do this. You don't *need* the cards, the crystals, the Yoni eggs, and the oils. If they feel good to use, use them. If you feel curious about them, try them. But don't be fooled that this is your answer to awakening. We don't need to go outside of ourselves to reveal ourselves to ourselves. What we need to do is to go inwards and get real and honest with ourselves.

THE RISE OF THE FEMININE

At the time of writing this book, the world is experiencing the pandemic that is Covid-19. In many ways humans are experiencing a giant pause, and an opportunity to reflect on our ways of living, how our lives are structured individually and as a collective, and what we value. This giant pause, I believe, is an opportunity for the continued rise of the feminine that we have been witnessing over many years. The rise of the feminine is about embracing and expressing of all parts of this energy; the powerful, fierce, and creative feminine as well as the soft, gentle, and nurturing feminine. The rise of the feminine is about moving in a direction that values life and celebrates what it is to really be alive by living in a way that is vibrant, expressive, creative, and full, rather than living in a way that focuses on productivity, and seeking and striving for more, no matter the cost. The rise of the feminine invites us back to simplicity and to live in connection to our Earth, to ourselves, and each other. The feminine embraces a creative and expansive mindset that looks for new ways of doing things rather than doing things the way they have always been done, and has a deep and full appreciation for our bodies, the meaning that we find in living, and the uniqueness of each individual that is to be celebrated along with our commonalities that unite us as human beings. The rise of the feminine invites an awareness of our duality, where things seem to be opposing, yet they are so deeply interconnected that they cannot be separated from one another. The rise of the feminine helps us to see all of the life that we were unable to see when we have an unbalanced and distorted overly masculine view of life.

Coronavirus has given us a great opportunity to see what it is like when the world embraces a slower-paced lifestyle that calls us to connect back to simplicity. It is nourishing for our people and our planet. We see people connecting back to simpler ways of living, and our planet replenishing itself. We have seen opportunities for new and innovative ways of doing things, like supported homeschooling in masses that would have otherwise been considered impossible. We have seen that we are capable of living a very different life, changing ways of being, and challenging the norm in no time at all. At the same time, we have witnessed how uncomfortable it feels for many people to have the luxuries of life being stripped away to a point where we are left only with ourselves to sit with. We have felt how uncomfortable it can be when we can offer ourselves little distraction from our lives through *doing*, and how uncomfortable it can feel to simply *be*. We can sense how much resistance we have to change when our lives are tipped upside down and we no longer have the control of our life that we thought we did. We begin to see how we do have control over all aspects of our life, and how much choice we have handed over to others.

Interestingly, at the same time that our perception of control is shattered, we are gifted an opportunity to look at our life and see where we have been choosing to live out of alignment with our true values. Losing a job that you rely on for income doesn't seem fair, but at the same time losing a job that you despised also creates an opportunity for one to look at how they might choose to create their life differently. I appreciate too that for many this time has been extremely challenging, and by no means am I saying that it is wrong to feel that. I myself found living in Melbourne at the time of extreme lockdown so intense that we decided to move back to North

Queensland where the impact of the virus was almost non-existent. Moving interstate, with 2 children, during a pandemic, whilst pregnant wasn't easy! The point I am trying to make is that in many ways we are seeing how uncomfortable it is when we invite a new way of being, and allow more feminine energy into our lives as individuals and as a whole.

At first, embracing the new ways of being feels foreign and pushes us to new edges. At the same time, we are gifted with an opportunity to access our creativity and to see how capable and resourceful we are as human beings. When we tip things on their head, and when we even up the imbalance of the parts of ourselves that we have suppressed we grow into something more beautiful than we could imagine.

In many ways, our attempts to give rise to the feminine have taken a counterintuitive masculine approach: "Hold your head high!", "Women can do anything!" "Women are equal to men!" Yes, we are! I completely agree but I feel, however, that where we have lost our footing in uplifting feminine is in our collective approach, by conforming to the masculine patriarchal lifestyle. A feminine approach to revealing our power and equality would embrace our inherent ways of being and invite more of our feminine energy than we currently do. This looks and feels so different to continuing to follow and use the patriarchal approach that we as a society have become accustomed to. Holding our head high wouldn't look like hiding our emotions and crying in the bathroom on our lunch break. It would mean embracing our emotions. "Women can do anything" wouldn't mean we have to push ourselves to do everything. Instead of working harder, trying to be more productive, and grinding though the days of our life, we would find ourselves *being more* and *bringing more of ourselves* to our life, being more creative, more vulnerable, more honest, more real, and living more of our truth. When we bring more of ourselves to our life, and when we allow ourselves to be more fully expressed in our truth and our values, we feel more ease and fulfilment.

This is the difference between *acting* capable, resilient, strong and resourceful, and *being* these things. When we feel like we need to act capable/resilient/strong/resourceful we believe we need to suppress parts of ourselves to fit a certain image. When we truly sense our capacity, our capability, our resourcefulness, and our strength, we can offer ourselves the level of self-acceptance that is required for us to reveal our full selves courageously and vulnerably. Pretending not to have particular emotions, needs, feelings, or desires is not what makes us equal, strong and powerful. It's the exact opposite. Feeling your emotions, acknowledging and meeting your needs, recognising your value, fulfilling your desires...*that* is what makes you strong, resilient, and capable. You do you, in your most unique way, in full self-expression, *that's* what the rise of the feminine is about.

EMBRACING YOUR FEMININE DOES NOT MEAN SUPPRESSING YOUR MASCULINE

Some would have you believe that embracing your feminine means you need to give up parts of yourself and personality that others might describe as masculine. I know that, for myself, when I first started exploring what it meant to embrace my feminine, I began to feel like parts of me were 'wrong', such as my love of running and weightlifting. What I know now is that these are simply things that I love, and that subduing these parts of me wasn't a way of embracing my feminine, it was just another way of criticising myself and trying to make myself fit into a mould that wasn't me! Fierce strength, resilience, and power are often mistaken as masculine qualities, when in fact they are the fire that burns within the feminine.

It's the dance between the masculine and feminine energies and the balance between them (ebb and flow, not equal parts always) that creates a sense of ease in our creative expression. Think of Mother Nature and all of her qualities. Sometimes she is dark, loud, and forceful, but she is not *always* that way. These qualities live within her and are part of her pulsating power. They are welcome and required for her to create in a way that allows her delicate ecosystem to exist. This is how I imagine the feminine within. She is strong, determined, powerful, resilient, and capable, but she channels her energy in such a way that does not disrupt her delicate ecosystem. She doesn't overwork, grind it out, or press on in times of exhaustion. Instead, she recognises what she needs to sustain her and to keep her well-nourished. She answers that call with whatever action or inaction may be required. She detects this from moment to moment, using the workings of her inner world to direct her movements in her outer world.

Embracing your feminine is not about fitting a mould by, for example, being more delicate. Embracing your femininity is about revealing more parts of yourself and nourishing your needs. My love of running and weightlifting isn't wrong or unfeminine. Feeling like I had to fit in my training at all costs and push myself to my limits constantly to feel some kind of self-worth felt out of balance for me. Embracing my feminine was not about stopping the intense movement, but more about allowing my movement practices to evolve to invite more variety (to allow for some slower, less intense movement), more mindfulness, and more opportunity for rest when it felt required.

To live comfortably in our skin is to embrace the dynamic and vast nature of the feminine, to know and speak our truth, and to express our self from the core of our being. When we have an understanding of our body and its natural rhythm we can begin to move from our centre. Moving from our centre physically, emotionally, and spiritually helps us to reveal more of our truth, which is the essential energetic medicine that helps us to feel whole. Through an understanding of and by connecting to the feminine aspects of our deep core, our pelvic floor, our womb space, and our menstrual cycle we begin to utilise our body's medicine. In the following chapters, you will access a better understanding of your body and the practices that will help you to embody this wisdom.

FEMININE CONNECTION AND
REFLECTION PRACTICES

Here are some simple reflective questions to help you become curious about how you feel about being female and how you sense the feminine within. You may find some of these answers quite revealing.

- What does being female mean to me?
- What does my feminine energy look and feel like?
- Where have I become disconnected from my feminine energy?
- Where have I become disconnected from my feminine body?
- If I was to step more into my feminine energy what would that look/feel like?
- How would I like to express my feminine energy?
- If I was to express my feminine energy more fully, how do I imagine my life would look/be/feel different?
- How do I feel about my pelvic health?
- Do I ignore pelvic health concerns? Why?
- How do I tend to my pelvic health?

- When I tune into the energy of my Pelvic Bowl, what is present for me?
- What aspects of my feminine body do I feel:
  - Disconnected to?
  - Shame around?
  - Inconvenienced by?
- What aspects of my feminine body do I:
  - Celebrate?
  - Feel a deep sense of connection to?
  - Embrace?
- If I was to embrace my feminine essence, honour my pelvic bowl, and tend to my pelvic health in a way that feels connected & celebrates being a woman:
  - What would that look like?
  - How would that feel?
  - What would I do more of?
  - What would I stop doing?

3

MENSTRUAL MAGIC

EMBRACING YOUR CYCLE

Imagine a world where instead of being taught that their body was radically inconvenient, women were supported in living in tune with their natural rhythm, the way nature intended!

As young women, many of us are taught that our cycle is embarrassing, that it should be kept secret, and that our blood is dirty. Think back to when you first got your period. Was it something to hide? Or was it celebrated? How do you feel about it now? Do you embrace your bleed or feel inconvenienced by it? Consider how we refer to menstrual health products as hygiene and sanitary items as if our period is dirty and unhygienic. I remember once staying at my boyfriend's (now husband's) place and leaving a box of tampons in the bathroom. I remember how his housemate exclaimed how gross it was to have left them there, like they were dirty and embarrassing and like I should have made a lot more effort to sneak them from my handbag to the toilet, holding each tampon tightly in my fist so that no one would see like I usually would. I'd become way too comfortable. My reaction when I got my first period was thinking that my time as a gymnast had expired. The sensation that my body was changing beyond my control felt awkward. Experimenting with tampons for the first time was physically and emotionally uncomfortable. Not knowing when my period would come again was scary. I imagined getting my period at school one day and finding blood all over my uniform because that had happened to a girl back in grade five. I remember how the entire grade was talking about it and how embarrassed I felt for her. Is this the way we want things to stay? Or could we imagine something different?

What if we were to show women that their natural rhythm is profoundly intelligent and progressive? What if we were to teach women that it was safe to accept and embrace their body, and to work *with* her body's energy and her natural ebb and flow, rather than pushing against it? What if we stopped making women feel like they are too soft and not tough enough to push through? What if rather than popping the pills and getting on with it, we could lean into our natural rhythm, and learn from its profound intelligence and capacity to create abundantly? I used to believe this was impossible. That there was simply no chance that in this productivity-driven world that this could one day be the case until I took radical personal responsibility for my life, my lifestyle, my choices, and my actions. Back then I used to believe that 'to keep on keeping on' was the only way forward but I realise now that that's a ticket to burnout, fatigue, loss of creativity, and a hugely unsustainable energetic investment.

Having tried and tested working *with* the rhythm of my body and embracing my cycle I now see that it starts with me. By embracing my cycle and my natural rhythm, not only do I lead a more nourishing, soul stimulating, and ease-filled life, I also get to share the flow-on effect with my children. We talk about my menstrual cycle openly in an age-appropriate way. I honour my need to rest when required and use my fertile force to create when I can. I work with my energy, not against it. I endeavour to teach my children to do the same. These small shifts create a profound impact over time.

SHAMEFUL, DIRTY, AND INCONVENIENT

Shameful, dirty, and inconvenient - this is how many women feel about their period, often without even realising it. I never knew that I thought that my period was dirty, until I realised that I did. It felt odd to realise because it was one of those times where you can suddenly see clearly that you believed something, not because you truly believed it for yourself, but because you had been taught to think that way. I realised I had a sense of shame about my period through my growing interest in creating more sustainable living practices and started questioning menstrual products and my choices. I'd always used tampons because I found pads too bulky and uncomfortable and I was considering a more sustainable option. I didn't want to use a menstrual cup, because I was concerned about the pressure it can create on the pelvic floor. The other option was reusable period underwear. My initial thoughts were that they would be *too dirty, too messy, and a bit yuck.* This is when I realised that I associated my period blood with being dirty.

What I find interesting about this is, before working as a pelvic floor physiotherapist, I was a cardiorespiratory physio in a hospital setting. What this meant was that I was very comfortable with all kinds of bodily fluids even when they weren't my own. I was comfortable holding vomit bags for patients when they were being sick, assisting elderly patients with pad changes, asking patients to cough up sputum, and taking a look at it to see how much they were able to cough up and how thick it was. The thought of this kind of work has some people's stomachs churning. How odd that I was so comfortable with this, and yet here I was concerned that my period blood was gross! I find it interesting too that, because of my pelvic health journey, I was very comfortable with using support pessaries, vaginal weights, doing internal pelvic massage with therapy wands etc. I didn't bat an eyelid at any of these things because they were serving functional purposes to help me build strength, relax my pelvic floor and gain support for the activities that I love like running and weightlifting. Here I am, very comfortable with all kinds of different vaginal products, comfortable doing internal pelvic therapy for myself and clients, and comfortable with all kinds of bodily fluids – yet the thought of cleaning underwear that had my menstrual blood on it seemed gross. Women's body shame is often like that. We don't realise how affected by body shame we are until we become more curious, and then we begin to see all the ways our shame hides beneath the surface. As soon as I tried the period pants, I realised that I didn't find my period blood gross or dirty at all. It was that I had learned that I should think that it was gross.

My connection to my cycle has deepened significantly over time and I now see it as a normal healthy part of me, and my body's natural state. I'm not ashamed to talk about my period. I don't feel burdened by my period and I embrace all of the different ways that I feel during different parts of my cycle, whether that be tired and in need of rest, reflection, and restoration, or energised, active, and more creative. How I feel in my body since embracing my cycle is worlds apart from when I felt my period was something to hide and that my blood was dirty. I feel at home.

I use the phases of my cycle to help me to understand why it is that I might feel a certain way. Instead of finding a fix, I give myself permission to simply feel how I do. I let myself slow down during my bleed time if/when I need to, and use it as an opportunity to reflect on what I would like to shed and let go of in my life. I now see my cycle as a part of me that I can connect to in order to understand my inner landscape, and something that I get to create ritual around. Knowing my cycle has gifted me a clear and tangible way of sensing my body's natural rhythm and cyclical nature, which helps me to be more kind and gentle with myself.

MEDICATION MASKING

Many women begin masking their menstrual cycle with medications at a young age. Young women are often prescribed contraceptive medications without much consideration for possible side effects. Often the reason for the pill is not for contraception itself, but rather for things like acne, period pain, or an attempt to 'control' an irregular cycle. Rather than giving our body time to find its natural rhythm, and time to go through some of the associated changes of puberty, our society yet again wrongs the female body, which leads many young women and their well-intending mothers to believe that the contraceptive pill/contraceptive medication is the answer.

I know for myself the reason I began using the pill was that my skin was 'out of control' and I needed something to 'fix' it. When I started using the pill I put on weight. When I put on weight my eating became disordered. I had bulimic tendencies - bingeing and purging. To help, my doctor prescribed antidepressants. They made me feel ill, but they did help me to stop my bulimic behaviours. Eventually, I weaned myself off the antidepressants and even though I had stopped the bingeing and purging, I still had a strained relationship with my body. I played with all kinds of diets and diet pills, none of which ever made a positive difference to how I felt in my skin. I don't blame the use of the pill for the lack of love that I had for my body back then, but it is certainly *one* of the *constant reminders* our society seems to unknowingly embrace that reinforces the message to women that our body is wrong in some way.

After the pill, I found Implanon. I liked it because I hardly got my period, which felt very convenient. I continued using the Implanon up until I was engaged. I chose to stop using all forms of hormonal contraception because I wanted to let my body rest before trying for a family. I was one of the lucky women whose cycle returned quickly after stopping hormonal contraception and it was only when I began thinking about starting a family that I learned that many women struggle with their cycle after using hormonal contraception.

Often, it's not until women stop using contraception as they plan for a family that they realise how severely it has affected their body. Some women who've been skipping their period for years, or who attributed their symptoms of amenorrhoea (absence of a menstrual period) with their contraceptive believing that their period would simply return once ceasing the medication, are shocked and disappointed when their period doesn't return as expected. As a society we accept that the contraceptive pill is a widely used drug, and take little time to consider the side effects, even though there is evidence that side effects of the pill can include:

- Hormonal confusion: missing or irregular periods, short cycles, infertility
- Digestive problems
- Energy reduction and symptoms of fatigue
- Skin changes, weight gain, and hair loss
- Mood disruption, including depression and anxiety
- Low libido, vaginal dryness, chronic vaginal infections, and pain with sex
- An increased risk of blood clots and stroke, breast, cervical and liver cancers, and diabetes. (Brighton, 2019)

The use of contraceptive medication is not wrong but the lack of information that women receive around the use and potential risks of contraceptive medications is a problem. The lack of choice that some women feel around the use of contraceptive medication is also hugely concerning.

In my conversations with women, it's not uncommon for women to say things like, "I've been told to use this contraception by my GP, and I would prefer not to be using any hormonal contraception, but he/she said I should, and so I am..." I remember meeting a GP for the first time after I had relocated to Melbourne and she asked me what I was using for contraception. When I told her that condoms were our preferred choice, she quickly steered the conversation towards using something more 'effective' like an IUD. Being strong in my values and well informed in my decisions around contraception, I simply said that I didn't want to consider any hormonal contraception and that I was very happy with my contraception choices.

Have you made an autonomous decision regarding contraception and hormonal medication?

It is disturbing how many women are using medications and contraceptive devices that they report cause significant discomfort, unwanted side effects and disagree with their body and their personal values, simply because a medical professional told them they should. I've seen countless examples of this, from the woman who shares with me, "I just don't like the thought of it," to the woman who says, "I was in excruciating pain all weekend, but the doctor told me to just give it more time to settle". Some women are prescribed contraceptive medication to improve period symptoms such as heavy bleeding or pain and often they tell me that they have felt absolutely no benefit from using it, but continue with its use because they don't feel like they have any other option. The body is sending clear messages, but women feel uncomfortable for listening to their instincts. Interestingly though, when given the opportunity to tune into their body, and when they ask themselves direct questions like, "What would you like to do?" or "What feels right for you and your body?" women are very capable of tapping into their body's awareness and saying: "Not using it anymore". We need to simply ask ourselves better questions and know that this is our body and therefore what we use for medication and contraception is our choice. You deserve to take an active role in deciding what contraception measures you take – whether they are for contraception or any other reason.

WHY TAKE NOTICE OF YOUR CYCLE

Living in a results-driven world that values productivity, it can seem like we don't have time to bleed. We don't have time to bleed, and we don't have time for all that's associated with having a rhythm and a cycle – the need for rest, recovery, and restoration. Ignoring our cycle and making attempts to dull it down or switch it off are further examples of how we disconnect from our body and our natural nature. It's the perfect example of how we devalue the female body, rather than embracing our feminine essence. What if, rather than being a burden, this natural cycle could be appreciated for the phenomenal wisdom that it holds and represents? The female body is dynamic, fluid, and cyclical. Yet we force ourselves to conform to the structure, rigidity, and a constant striving that leads us to end up feeling depleted, exhausted, and uninspired.

We all know that feeling when we've lost our flow and our rhythm, when we just need to walk away from something because no matter how hard we try things aren't progressing in a positive direction. When we get that feeling though, how often do we stop and let ourselves walk away? How often do we let our energy be utilised in a way that feels more resonant and more valuable? Now consider how often we press on because it's expected? Either we expect it of ourselves, or someone else expects it of us. We press on because that's just the way things are done, even though we know that it's a waste of time, energy, and effort.

Pressing on in times where rest, reflection, restoration, and recovery are required is what many of us do. Even though our body screams for rest, our creative energy feels zapped, and life in general feels like such a grind that we keep on going because it's expected. We also get glimpses of what happens when we do walk away from something and come back some other time. Our energy feels restored, our creativity explodes, and we find the rhythm and the flow again. This is the opportunity we have when we choose to work *with* our rhythm of our body and our cycle. When we choose to drop our internal expectations of having to be on all the time and when we can take full ownership of how we create our life, we can choose to move with the rhythm of our cycle and find the ease and the flow that accompanies our natural rhythm.

Nature is infinitely intelligent, and our menstrual cycle shows quite clearly that we are designed to flow in a rhythm. You just need to consider the seasons or notice how a flower reseeds itself to appreciate how valuable the natural cycles of nature are. It offers the much-needed time for rest before another phase of regeneration and growth begins. When we can tap into our body we can harness and work with its energy, rather than working against it. It's our human brain that tries to manipulate our circumstances and perceives our body's timing as inconvenient. It stops us from accessing our powerful, natural, internal rhythm that we so desire. When we stop with the hustle and grind, we get to sense the ease of the rhythm. This is what tuning into your cycle is all about.

Perhaps the best first step towards tuning into your cycle is understanding what a healthy cycle looks and feels like.

THE FEMALE REPRODUCTIVE SYSTEM

The female reproductive system is located in the central compartment of the pelvis and is comprised of the upper reproductive tract and the lower reproductive tract. The upper reproductive tract includes two ovaries, two fallopian tubes, and the uterus (AKA the womb). The vagina makes up the lower reproductive tract. In 'normal' anatomy women have two oval-shaped ovaries, one on each side of the uterus. They are approximately 3cm x 1.5cm x 1.5cm. The main role of the ovaries is egg maturation and hormonal secretion during a standard menstrual cycle.

THE FEMALE REPRODUCTIVE SYSTEM

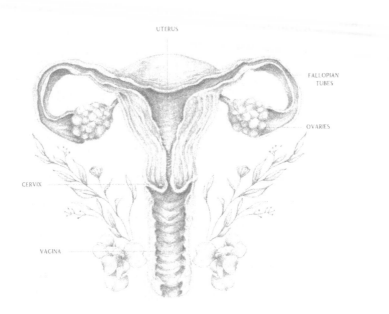

The uterus is an upside-down pear-shaped muscular organ, normally the size of an adult fist. Its functional purpose is mechanical protection, nutritional support, and waste removal for a developing embryo/foetus. The muscular contraction of the uterus is what helps to move baby through the birth canal at the time of delivery. The uterus consists of three main parts: the fundus, the body, and the cervix. The cervix contains the channel leading to the vagina and is the part of the uterus that we may feel when we insert a finger into the vagina.

WHAT DOES A HEALTHY CYCLE LOOK LIKE?

The *average* menstrual cycle is regarded as 28 days in length but a *normal* menstrual cycle can range from anywhere between 21-35 days in length. This timeframe is defined as starting from the first day (Day 1) of the menstrual bleed, through to the last day before the next menstrual bleed (Day 21-35).

The menstrual cycle is divided into halves with the days up to ovulation being the follicular phase and the days after ovulation are the luteal phase.

Women vary in their bleed time from around three days up to seven days. A bleed time longer than seven days is considered to be prolonged bleeding. (Cuss and Abbott, 2014)

Ovulation occurs around mid-cycle. It is generally accepted that during the average woman's menstrual cycle there are six days when intercourse can result in pregnancy. This fertile window comprises the five days before ovulation and the day of ovulation itself. However, it's important to know that this can vary from woman to woman, and from cycle to cycle.

The second phase of the cycle is called the luteal phase. It is the luteal phase that is the standard phase. As a general rule, the luteal phase lasts 14 days. Ovulation, therefore, occurs 14 days before the start of the next period.

The main reproductive hormones that fluctuate throughout the menstrual cycle are oestrogen, progesterone, and luteinising hormone (LH).

There is a surge of oestrogen and LH around ovulation to help release the egg from the ovary. After that point, oestrogen generally drops but will rebuild somewhat to help to build the uterine lining.

Progesterone (PRO gestation) is more dominant in the second half of the cycle.

Progesterone helps to relax the smooth muscle of the uterus, preventing uterine contractions if there is a foetus developing. Progesterone also helps to control the degree of growth of the uterine lining. Around day 28, if there is no developing foetus, progesterone drops and a period will occur.

MENSTRUAL CYCLE

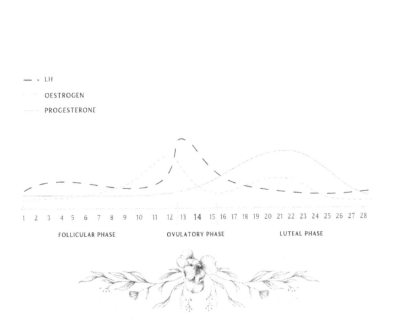

NORMAL MENSTRUAL BLOOD LOSS

Normal menstrual blood loss is between 30-40mls per period with a range between 10-80mls. More than 80mls is considered to be heavy menstrual blood loss. The number of sanitary items used is a poor predictor of menstrual blood loss as many women change their hygiene products out of convenience rather than need. The following markers, however, are considered relevant:

- Soaking through one or more sanitary pads/tampons items every hour for several hours
- Needing to use double sanitary protection
- Needing to wake more than once through the night to change sanitary protection
- Needing to restrict activities due to menstrual flow
- Symptoms of anaemia such as tiredness, fatigue, or shortness of breath (Cuss and Abbott, 2014)

If you sense that you have abnormal uterine bleeding it is recommended that you seek medical advice. If you do seek medical advice, I encourage you to find a practitioner who will listen to you, and work with you to find out what may be the underlying cause. Masking the problem with medication doesn't fix the problem, and often creates a deeper disconnect with our body. Using medication to treat symptoms isn't necessarily wrong or bad, but I urge you to give yourself time to make conscious decisions around how you approach managing abnormal bleeding.

CONNECT TO THE RHYTHM OF YOUR CYCLE

Our menstrual cycles often follow a particular rhythm. When you begin to tune into your cycle, you will likely begin to notice patterns emerge in relation to your emotional state, your energy levels, and how you feel in your body in general. Some of this may be consistent with the experiences of other women and some unique to you. We can look to the seasons and moon phases to help give us some understanding of these rhythms and patterns.

When we look at the phases of the moon, we can see its consistencies and similarities to the menstrual cycle. It has four main phases including the New Moon, Waxing Moon, Full Moon, and the Waning Moon. It runs on a 28-day cycle, similar to the menstrual cycle. When we tune into the moons energy we can sense a similar pattern to that of the menstrual cycle energy. New moon or 'Dark Moon' energy is similar to that of our menstrual bleed energy. It is a reflective and releasing energy, and a time to connect with new intentions and new desired ways of being. The Waxing Moon has a similar energy to the follicular phase of our cycle, with building energy and increasing momentum. The Full Moon, radiant, bright, and full of heightened energy and activity, is similar to the energy of ovulation. Finally, the Waning Moon is similar to that of the luteal phase, where we draw our energy inward and move back into rest mode. Although we can draw these similarities, not all women will feel the need to rest and restore during their bleed time, just as some women won't feel radiant during ovulation at times. Some women talk of Period Power – a sense of surging energy on during their period. I myself used to feel this. It was like a release of building tension within, physically and emotionally. My body would want to run after a time of needing more rest on the days leading up to my period. Nowadays, I feel more of a need to rest and restore around my bleed time. This is an important point too, that our body changes over time, and how we feel during different phases of our cycle can change over time too.

Though there are similarities in the lunar energy cycle and the menstrual cycle, it doesn't mean that we will necessarily bleed during a New Moon and ovulate at the Full Moon. Sometimes this may be the case, and depending on your cycle it is likely to shift and change over time. It's certainly not wrong to bleed during the Full Moon, and ovulate at the New Moon, and trying to 'sync' our cycle to fit the lunar phases is just another way that we can ignore our body. A far more powerful thing to try is simply noticing how we are feeling, and tuning into the energy of our body. When we can do that, and honour that, we can notice the patterns that emerge but we don't find ourselves trying to control our body and forcing ourselves to feel something that we don't.

I certainly believe that the moon phase can affect how we feel and of course, our menstrual cycle affects how we feel. Probably not in equal amounts, and sometimes more than others. Being fluid and flexible, being able to sense how you feel and respond to your body's energy is what connects you to your cycle. When we try to take a rigid and controlling approach toward connecting to our cycle, and when we find that we are wronging our body for how it feels, we know we have stepped away from this connection.

The rhythm of the menstrual cycle can be likened to other natural cycles, in particular, the lunar cycle and the seasons. In the following pages, I share some of these energetic similarities. As you begin to take notice of your cycle, there are a few key questions that you may like to consider.

You may wish to create a simple journal that follows the days of your cycle, beginning on day one of your bleed and recording the answers to the following questions:

- *How am I feeling physically in my body?*
- *How do I feel emotionally?*
- *How do I feel energetically?*
- *What would feel nourishing?*

Once you have tracked your cycle for about 3-6 months you will likely begin to notice some patterns in how you feel physically, emotionally, and energetically at different phases of your cycle. You may have an idea of how long to expect your bleed to continue and how it acts in terms of heaviness and flow, you may also determine when you are ovulating and the phases that fall either side.

Menstruation
Days 1 – 7(ish)

Bleed time
New Moon / Dark Moon
Wintertime Energy – inward and reflective
Releasing and letting go of anything that no longer serves you

How you *may* feel:

- Requiring more rest and spaciousness in your life
- Less like being social and 'on'
- Reflective and contemplative
- Less active, wanting to connect with slower-paced movement
- Wanting to engage less with people who are not part of your inner sacred circle

MENSTRUAL CYCLE RHYTHM

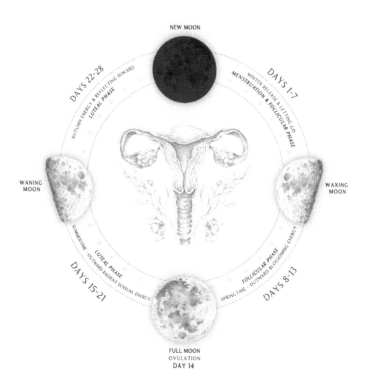

NEW MOON

DAYS 22-28
AUTUMN ENERGY & REFLECTING INWARD
LUTEAL PHASE

DAYS 1-7
WINTER RELEASE & LETTING GO
MENSTRUATION & FOLLICULAR PHASE

WANING
MOON

WAXING
MOON

SUMMERTIME · OUTWARD RADIENT SENSUAL ENERGY
LUTEAL PHASE
DAYS 15-21

FOLLICULAR PHASE
SPRINGTIME · OUTWARD BLOSSOMING ENERGY
DAYS 8-13

FULL MOON
OVULATION
DAY 14

There may be a tendency to want to skip this phase of your cycle because it asks us to slow down and come inward. When we are feeling inconvenienced by our cycle, particularly our bleed time, common practices are to pop a pill to mask our symptoms, drink more coffee or stimulants, and eat more sugar in an attempt to keep our energy up. Surrendering to the slower pace, nurturing and nourishing your body and using this time to rest and restore is how we can tap into the power of our cycle so that we are ready to take action in a new phase with more ease.

Examples of lifestyle choices that women make in response to this phase of their cycle:

- Booking fewer clients or arranging less intense workloads
- Choosing to work from home instead of the office
- Making fewer social commitments
- Choosing walking over running, Yin yoga over Vinyasa flow, lighter weights over heavier ones etc.
- Some research shows greater strength gains with resistance training during this phase of your cycle but this is also the time where some women will feel increased pelvic symptoms such as prolapse and incontinence. Tune into your body. If you feel you have 'period power' you may like to use this phase in your cycle for strength training. If you experience pelvic symptoms, lighter weights and reduced intensity of exercise is recommended.
- Taking time to reflect on what no longer serves you and practicing release ritual/s like journaling/freewriting about what you wish to let go of and perhaps burning the paper afterward or burying it into the ground to return this energy to the earth to create space for new seeds to be planted and nourished.

Follicular
Days 8 – 13(ish)

Pre-ovulation, Follicular phase
Waxing Moon
Springtime energy - outward blossoming
Focused, driven, social, creative, active

How you *may* feel in your body:

- Increasing energy, vitality, and clarity
- Effervescent creative energy: a yearning to start or continue creative projects with newfound vitality and clarity (this may build over time)
- Wanting to move your body in more expressive ways with building energy, strength, and stamina

Examples of lifestyle choices that women make in response to this phase of their cycle:

- Reengaging with creative projects
- Planning for meetings, social events, and reconnecting with work colleagues/potential clients
- Doing more upbeat movement with a strong element of self-expression – perhaps dancing, flow yoga, or jogging

Ovulation + Luteal
Days 14 – 21(ish)

Ovulation Phase
Full Moon and Summertime Energy
Outward, radiant energy.

How you *may* feel in your body:

- More sensual, sexual, and radiant
- Wanting to be more social and connect with friends, family, partners
- Feeling your creativity blossom, wanting to share projects and creations

- Wanting to move your body in more energetic ways and wanting to connect with nature through movement practices

Examples of lifestyle choices that women make in response to this phase of their cycle:

- Connecting with friends and being more social
- Booking in more clients and heading into the office
- Doing more and utilising your increased energy and vitality
- Engaging in conversations/situations where you want to feel confident, energetic, and charismatic

Luteal
Days 22-28(ish)

Pre-Menstruation Luteal Phase
Waning Moon
Autumn Energy – reflective, inward

How you *may* feel

- Reflective and contemplative
- In a 'pruning' phase - deciding what is not necessarily, preparing for release
- Taking time to come back down in your energy, engaging with slower movement
- Taking more time for rest and recovery, and craving more spaciousness in your days
- Connecting with those in your inner circle, and winding down your social activity

HOW TO TUNE INTO YOUR UNIQUE RHYTHM

There are numerous ways you can tune into and track your cycle. Some women use a traditional calendar, some use apps, and some use moon cycle charts. It's completely up to you what feels resonant and good and there are a couple of things that I recommend you be aware of when you do start to tune into your cycle.

When it comes to tracking your cycle- in particular how you feel during different phases of your cycle- remember that it is open to change. Our menstrual cycle has a huge impact on our energy, our emotions and how we feel in our physical body - but it's not *the ONLY thing* that impacts how we feel. Bringing awareness to your cycle can be profoundly powerful, but even more powerful is to simply tune in to your body on a more frequent basis. While we will notice some patterns and rhythm to how we feel during the different phases of our cycle, there will be some changes that we can't predict. This doesn't mean you're tracking your cycle incorrectly, or that you're doing something wrong, it means that your body is fluid and always changing.

Whilst there are some excellent systems out there that will help you to track your cycle, I recommend that you choose wisely. Some systems will try to tell you how you *will* or *should* feel at each phase of your cycle. While in some ways this can be useful, I don't believe anyone can tell you how you will/should feel at any particular phase in your cycle. That would require you to hand over our power to someone else living outside of your body. Only you can know how you feel at any particular moment and you cannot get that wrong. Trust your body and your experience.

THE IMPACT OF THE MENSTRUAL CYCLE
ON PELVIC ORGAN PROLAPSE
AND INCONTINENCE SYMPTOMS

As mentioned earlier, the two main hormones that fluctuate during the menstrual cycle are oestrogen and progesterone. As the levels of these hormones change throughout our cycle, they can have an impact on pelvic organ prolapse (POP) symptoms and urinary incontinence. At times during our cycle when oestrogen is low (particularly on the days leading up to our period and during our period), symptoms of POP and incontinence can increase. Many women describe an increase in Pelvic Organ Prolapse symptoms (listed below) during this phase in their cycle.

- A 'bulging' sensation in the vagina
- A heaviness or dragging sensation within the pelvis
- Lower back pain
- Difficulty initiating/completing a bladder/bowel motion
- Incontinence or leakage from the bladder or the bowel
- Pain with sex (a deep thudding sensation)

Similarly, because of the changes in hormones during lactation, breastfeeding mothers may feel an improvement of prolapse or incontinence symptoms when their period returns indicating that their overall oestrogen levels have increased.

Some women wonder why they sometimes leak urine during particular activities, and other times don't – taking notice of their cycle and when their incontinence seems to be worse can help to explain this. Due to hormonal changes throughout their cycle, some women experience more leakage during menstruation and the days leading up to menstruation, others at ovulation.

Hormonal impacts, particularly during the luteal phase, can make the digestive system sluggish, meaning that bowel motility can slow down and can cause constipation. Constipation can cause prolapse symptoms to become worse as a result of the downward pressure on the pelvic floor when straining to use the bathroom. Incontinence symptoms may in fact be improved by the obstruction created by the stool. The stool creates pressure within the pelvis, which helps to maintain urethral closure – which stops leaking. This may sound desirable but is not ideal. To help maintain good pelvic health, decrease bloating and improve constipation, you may wish to increase the fibre in your diet during phases where progesterone is high – particularly in the luteal (second half) of your cycle.

MOVEMENT AND MENSTRUATION

Depending on their background and philosophy, some practitioners will recommend that women who experience significant period pain reduce the amount of exercise, particularly at the time of their period. Other wellness advocates will urge women to avoid higher intensity exercise altogether, implying that it is overly masculine and that it doesn't promote optimal wellbeing for women. I believe that honouring our personal value system has a huge impact on our wellbeing, and therefore honouring what is important to you as an individual will have better outcomes as opposed to being told what you should or shouldn't be doing with your body.

When it comes to movement and mensuration there are a few things to consider.

Firstly, what is important to you? If you are an athlete that is trying to achieve a personal best how you approach your movement, and what benefits you are hoping to gain from working with your menstrual cycle will be very different from a woman who moving simply for the pleasure of moving her body. In addition, it's important to consider if you have any pelvic concerns that would impact how you want to move your body. If you do, it may be helpful for you to know how exercise and movement impact your symptoms. For example, if you have symptoms of pelvic organ prolapse (p. 120 - 121), you may choose to decrease the intensity of your exercise during the bleed time when symptoms may become worse, whereas if you experience dysmenorrhea (pain with menstrual bleeding), increasing your exercise might help to reduce your pain. This is why blanket statements about what will feel good to you during different phases of your cycle are not helpful. You are individual and unique, and what feels good and when it feels good will be unique to you. That being said, some information may help to guide you as to how to choose to move your body during menstruation.

- There is some evidence to show that women experience *greater strength gains* with strength training during the *follicular phase* of their cycle. (Sung et al., 2014) However, this can also be the time when women experience greater pelvic stress symptoms such as pelvic organ prolapse (POP) and Stress Urinary Incontinence.
- *Oestrogen* is thought to *improve continence and POP symptoms*. At times of decreased oestrogen, particularly in the *follicular phase, symptoms of incontinence and POP can, therefore, become worse.*
- *Higher levels of progesterone in the luteal phase* can lead to constipation, and *worsen prolapse symptoms*. Increasing exercise can help to improve bowel motility. Therefore, if prolapse symptoms are worse during the second half of your menstrual

cycle, and you experience constipation, exercise may be more helpful than remaining inactive.

- Constipation can reduce incontinence because the obstruction of the stool acts as a 'backstop' for the bladder. If incontinence symptoms seem to improve during the luteal phase and you have constipation, you might think that your decreased symptoms are due to having changed something about your exercise regime, when it may be a direct result of constipation.

- For women who have *primary dysmenorrhea exercise has shown to have the largest effect in regards to reducing menstrual pain* compared to no treatment. Exercise has been demonstrated to be moderately more effective than analgesic medication and have a large reduction in pain compared to no treatment. Low-intensity exercise, consisting of yoga and stretching, showed the largest and most consistent positive benefit. (Armour et al., 2019)

- In a much smaller pilot study of women with primary dysmenorrhoea, it was demonstrated that aerobic exercise increased progesterone. New evidence is emerging to demonstrate that this increase in progesterone may ultimately lead to decreased uterine cramping and therefore reduce pain. Because this is such new information, we cannot say for sure but *it appears that aerobic exercise such as brisk walking may help to reduce pain in women who have primary dysmenorrhoea.* (Khannan et al., 2019)

- Women with *endometriosis* (a common yet frequently under-recognised chronic disease that occurs when cells similar to those that line a woman's uterus grow in other parts of her body, usually around the pelvis, and less commonly in tissues and organs outside the pelvic cavity) often experience what is considered secondary dysmenorrhoea (menstrual pain that is associated with an identifiable pathology, such as endometriosis). Unfortunately, at this point, there *is limited evidence* regarding secondary dysmenorrhoea and the physiological benefits of exercise. However, given that evidence is emerging to support exercise in the treatment of primary dysmenorrhoea, it is *promising that exercise may have a similar impact on secondary dysmenorrhoea.*

Having this information as you experiment with different types of exercises and noticing the impact it has at different phases of your cycle is the key to movement and menstruation. Becoming aware of how your body responds to exercise and adjusting your movement accordingly will be your best guide.

PRODUCT PREFERENCES

From my personal experience and through my work with other women I've certainly noticed a few things that change in terms of menstrual health product preferences when you begin to connect with and tune into your cycle. As you live more in touch with your natural cycle, you tend to connect more deeply to nature. When you connect more deeply to our Earth, you begin to become more aware of the environmental impact of your choices.

I'm not aware of any excellent high-quality studies that take feminine products head-to-head and measure their impact on the environment, but certainly, there is a growing choice around more sustainable menstrual products for women, like reusable period pants and menstrual cups. I wouldn't advocate for one choice over the other, but there are certainly a few things to consider when choosing sanitary items.

Menstrual Cups:

More women are choosing sustainable menstrual products and menstrual cups are a popular choice. They are eco-friendly, often comfortable, convenient, and work well. What women often don't know is how to remove them safely, which is imperative for pelvic health. Without safe removal, cups can create a direct downward pressure upon the pelvic floor which may lead to an increased risk of pelvic organ prolapse (POP) or an increase in symptoms of an existing POP.

To remove your cup safely, be sure to release the seal before gently pulling it from your vagina. You can do this by squeezing the bottom of the cup, or by inserting a finger to release the seal created by the rim of the cup. Before you remove the cup, you can also gently squeeze the pelvic floor muscles to provide some counteractive lift to the pulling of the cup.

For some women, menstrual cups may not be the best choice. It's your choice, and some women find them quite supportive (similar to a pessary). If you have an existing prolapse, I wouldn't say you shouldn't use cups but if you do find your symptoms become worse when you use a menstrual cup, I would suggest considering an alternative. If a cup just doesn't feel right, you don't need to feel the pressure to use one because it's more sustainable. There are fantastic alternatives - like period underwear and if they don't feel good remember that few of us are perfect in our environmental practices! You don't need to be afraid of cups, just mindful of how to use them and if they are right for you.

The second thing that I noticed for myself and other women regarding period products and creating a connection to their cycle is the desire to 'allow the flow', meaning that women begin to choose products that tend to allow the feeling of flow, rather than the restriction of it. In this case, pads or period underwear seem to be the preferred choice.

Tampons:

Some women find that after giving birth tampons don't seem to fit as comfortably as they once did. This is often due to the changes in the connective tissue and musculature of the pelvic floor. These changes can mean that the vaginal walls now have a different structure and perhaps more elasticity. Difficulty inserting or ill-fitting tampons that used to feel comfortable can be a symptom of Pelvic Organ Prolapse (though not always). If this concerns you, I encourage you to seek advice from a women's health physiotherapist. You will find more reading on pelvic health and POP in other chapters of this book.

Toilet Paper as a form of Menstrual Product:

I've had quite a few women tell me that their menstrual product preference is in fact toilet paper. They often begin their sentence with, "You probably think this is gross, but..." I don't think that using toilet paper for your period is 'wrong' or 'gross' or 'yucky'. It's simply a preference. If it's your preference, know that you are not alone and that your choice is not wrong.

MENSTRUAL HEALTH REFLECTIVE QUESTIONS

Here are some questions you may wish to consider to help you decide if you're content with your menstrual health and your connection to your cycle. Some relate to your connection to your cycle now, and some will reveal what has influenced your relationship with your cycle over time.

- What was my introduction to my cycle like? Was there openness, and celebration? Or was it thought to be shameful/dirty/something to be secretive about?
- How did my initiation to my cycle impact my relationship with my cycle and my body?
- What stories do I have about my menstrual cycle? Are they my own? If I was to choose a different narrative, what would it be?
- How do I experience my cycle now? Do I see it as inconvenient? How? Powerful? How?
- Is my body bringing my attention and awareness to my cycle in the form of pain?
- What is my body asking of me?
- Do I try and dull down my body's needs at different times of my cycle?
- Do I make conscious decisions around any medication I use to help me move through different phases of my cycle?
- Would I like to create more space around certain phases of my cycle to allow for rest?
- Does my current choice around the contraception I use reflect my values? Have I considered how this form of contraception impacts my body? Have I made this decision for myself, or have I let someone else make it for me?
- Does my current form of period product/s feel good and comfortable for me? Or would I prefer to be using something else? Does my body feel drawn to using something different?
- Do I expect my periods to be painful? Could it be possible for me to experience more comfort throughout my cycle? Have I accepted my pain to be 'normal' when it doesn't feel normal to me?

- If I've experienced a change in my cycle, does it feel like my body is asking for awareness and attention? Or does it feel like a normal shift - not wrong, just different?
- Do I allow myself to feel tired and more in touch with my emotional body throughout different phases of my cycle?
- Do I allow myself to tap into my natural rhythm and allow my life and lifestyle to reflect that?
- Or do I feel like I'm living up to the expectations of others?
- How do I feel about my cycle?
- How would I like to feel about my cycle?
- If I was to embrace my internal rhythm, what would I do? What would I stop doing?
- How is my body calling me to heal any shame associated with my menstrual cycle?

As you connect to your body's guidance you can create new practices and a new relationship with your cycle in a way that resonates with you.

4

HOLISTIC PELVIC HEALTH

THE DEEP CORE

Taking a whole-body integrated approach to pelvic health requires us to have an understanding of the anatomical and physiological deep core and pelvic floor, as well as an appreciation of the subtle energetic core. The purpose of this section is to help you gain a better understanding of your body and to provide some important links between our physical core and our energetic core.

Usually, when physiotherapists, movement coaches, personal trainers, etc. refer to the core, they are referring to your deep core. In its physical sense, I like to think of our deep core as our foundation for fitness, movement, and strength. Our deep core creates a stable base for us to move from.

The deep core is a group of *four muscles* in the shape of a canister.

- At the top is the **diaphragm,** the main muscle responsible for breathing mechanics
- At the bottom, the **pelvic floor.**
- At the front, the **transverse abdominis (TA)** the deepest abdominal muscle that wraps around our thorax like a corset
- At the back, our **multifidus** muscle offering deep spinal support

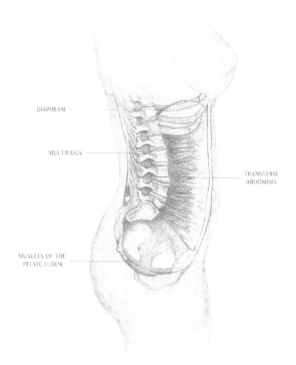

The deep core provides us with our central stability. Before we perform any task or movement, our deep core engages, acting as an anchor for our limbs. This is why I refer to our core as our foundation for fitness and movement. If the deep core does not work effectively, our foundation is compromised.

The deep core works as a pressure system. The muscles within the core are designed to work in a particular pattern to respond to changes in our intra-abdominal pressure as we prepare for and undertake any kind of movement. As we inhale the diaphragm descends, the pelvic floor relaxes and softens to allow for the change in pressure. Similarly, the abdominal muscles relax and bulge with each inhale. When we exhale, the pelvic floor gently lifts and recoils inwards and the transverse abdominis (TA) recoil, drawing the belly button towards the spine. We don't need to consciously create or force this muscle contraction, this is simply how our body moves with our breath. This natural movement is a beautiful reminder of our body's wisdom and how each of the components of our body works in harmony with one another. You can sense this in your own body using Part One of The Deep Core Connection Practice (p. 273 - 277).

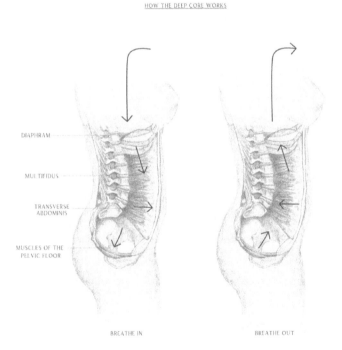

HOW THE DEEP CORE WORKS

DIAPHRAM

MULTIFIDUS

TRANSVERSE ABDOMINIS

MUSCLES OF THE PELVIC FLOOR

BREATHE IN   BREATHE OUT

THE PELVIC FLOOR

The *pelvic floor muscles* are a group of muscles that form a sling that creates the floor to our pelvic ring and the base of our pelvic bowl. The muscles of the pelvic floor attach from the pubic bone at the front, to the coccyx (tail bone) at the back, and to the ischial tuberosity (sit bones) on the left and right of the pelvis. There are two layers of muscles that make up the pelvic floor muscles; the deep pelvic floor muscular layer that makes up the internal muscles of the pelvic floor and the superficial layer that make up the external layer of the pelvic floor. The deep pelvic floor muscles are responsible for providing 'lift' to the pelvic organs and supporting the connective tissue of the pelvis. The superficial muscles help to give added closure to the vagina and the anus.

It's important to know that the pelvic floor in its entirety is *more than just muscles*. It is also made up of a complex network of sphincters that open and shut to initiate and stop bladder and bowel emptying, nerves, and ligaments, and fascia that provide support.

Physically the pelvic floor has a significant role in:

- Maintaining continence - stopping leakage from the bladder and bowel
- Sexual pleasure - orgasm
- Supporting the pelvic organs - the bladder, bowel, and uterus in place

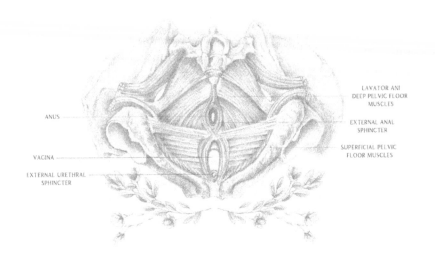

THE PELVIC FLOOR

LAVATOR ANI
DEEP PELVIC FLOOR
MUSCLES

ANUS

EXTERNAL ANAL
SPHINCTER

SUPERFICIAL PELVIC
FLOOR MUSCLES

VAGINA

EXTERNAL URETHRAL
SPHINCTER

THE ENERGETIC CORE

I think of the core as an energetic centre within our body. Essentially the energetic core is made up of our pelvic bowl, the female reproductive organs that sit within this bowl and the pelvic floor that supports it, our gut-brain (a place of intuition and personal power), our heart, and our lungs. Life force radiates from this space – our womb that creates life, our heart that keeps us alive, and our lungs that breathe life. This is the space in our body that holds the truth of who we are at the core of our being. Being in powerful communication with this space, therefore, helps us to create a life that feels aligned with our truth, our values, and who we are at our core.

Connecting to our deep core energy helps to:

- Keep us grounded
- Become aware when we step out of alignment
- Sense our self-worth and own our personal power
- Connect to our values, our dreams, and desires
- Connect to our feminine wisdom, our intuition, and our creativity
- Be open to life
- Connect to other human beings and our world with love, kindness, and respect
- Connect to the 'core' of who we are

There are many ways that we can access a deeper connection to our core energy. Connecting to your centre doesn't require anything particularly fancy, or esoteric. It simply requires intention and practice.

When we connect with our core, our body, and our feminine energy, we bring greater awareness to how we are crafting our life. When we open the door to accessing our core we open a door for positive change, deep self-connection, self-love, and self-discovery. We start to understand our natural nature and connect to our truth. We learn how changing simple aspects of how we approach our self and our life can create huge change over time. We see the interconnectedness of everything, and we take back responsibility and ownership of our body, our being, and our lives.

Understanding the muscles of the deep core and their function helps us to understand the more subtle energy body and what it represents.

THE PELVIC BOWL

The pelvis consists of three bones, the left and right hip bones, and the sacrum. These bones form a ring. The circular ring of the pelvis and the underlying muscles of the pelvic floor create the pelvic bowl. On a physical level, the pelvic bowl houses the female reproductive organs, as well as the bladder and the bowel. This physical space in the female body is a powerful creative centre. Not only is it where life is created, but it is also the fertile ground in which all forms of creativity are seeded, fertilised, nurtured, grown, and birthed.

This powerful centre of a woman's body is also the space that holds the key to immense pleasure, not only of a sexual nature, but the simple pleasure that comes from experiencing the powerful connection we have with other women, our children, and nature itself.

Throughout our lifetime, women are consistently brought back to this space in their bodies. From the beginning of menstruation, we are gifted a cyclical reminder of our natural rhythm and our connection to Mother Earth. Through pregnancy, miscarriage, birth, sex, and menopause, our attention is drawn to this space over and over again throughout our lifetime. Women who live in tune with their body, in particular the pelvic space, know that this is no mistake.

THE PELVIS

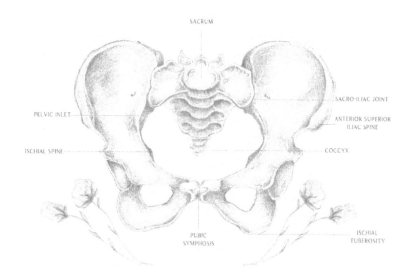

SACRUM

SACRO-ILIAC JOINT

PELVIC INLET

ANTERIOR SUPERIOR
ILIAC SPINE

ISCHIAL SPINE

COCCYX

PUBIC
SYMPHOSIS

ISCHIAL
TUBEROSITY

PELVIC ENERGY

You can see that from a physical standpoint, the pelvic floor has an important role in offering us *support*. Being the floor to the pelvic bowl, it has an intricate relationship to all that is housed within our pelvic bowl, in particular our female reproductive organs including our uterus/womb - our physical creative centre that produces life. The pelvic floor, along with the uterus and ovaries, hold valuable information for us around our acceptance of our feminine body and our feminine energy, and all forms of our creativity.

As women, many of us have become disconnected from this space in our body due to societal suppression of feminine energy, and inherited belief systems such as 'creativity is not as important as productivity' or 'embracing your femininity is a sign of weakness'. Over many years women have disconnected from their feminine energy, and are now lacking in rituals and self-care practices that help us to honour this sacred space, particularly in the Western world.

Rather than reading about this space, feeling it for yourself is much more powerful. The Body Connection Practices (pages 266-298) section of this book contains a series of practices that you can use to help you connect with this space.

When we feel connected to this space in our body, we:

- Feel the power of our feminine energy
- Understand the value of living in tune with the ebb and flow of our cycle
- Create at a pace that allows for potency and ease, rather than pushing ourselves into overdrive and forcing ourselves to keep on keeping on
- Have clear, loving limits and boundaries in all of our relationships
- Have a healthy sexual desire and can express our desire openly and vulnerably in safe environments
- Can assert independent judgement
- Connect with others through grounded emotions
- Live with fluidity and trust in ourselves and our support networks
- Lean into the support of others and can sense the support that the universe offers to us always

When we are disconnected from this space, or when it is requiring some attention from us we:

- Feel burdened by our feminine body and our feminine nature. Our monthly cycle is inconvenient, our body is never good enough
- We feel like we are too much - too erratic, unstable, too emotional, too sensitive
- Lack healthy and clear boundaries in our relationships - in our sexual relationships, our friendships, our working relationships
- Feel an imbalance of our sexual desire – either it is lacking, or it feels like it's in overdrive
- We feel like our feminine body and anything related to it is taboo, dirty, or wrong in some way
- Lack independent judgement
- Have difficulty accepting support from others, and can feel like the world is against us more often than not

WOMB ENERGY

Our uterus or womb is a powerful, creative, and fertile centre of all forms of creativity – whether it be a book, a garden, or a way of mothering. When we live and create from this space, we do so in a way that is connected to both our feminine and masculine energy. Often, in our very masculine world, women and men find themselves creating in a way that is more reflective of masculine energy with little input from the feminine. When we create with an overly masculine tone we are constantly producing, have little space for inspiration to seed and grow, regard our inner knowing and intuition as inferior, and give ourselves limited allowance to rely on our foundational support systems.

For some women creating in a way that honours both the masculine and feminine energy requires a simple subtle awareness and is an already embodied practice. For other women, it can feel terrifying. The sound of rest, reflection, slowing down, waiting for inspiration to seed, and taking action when the time feels right seems so foreign and so unfamiliar that trusting in this way of creating seems ridiculous, scary, irrational, and irresponsible. This was exactly how I felt when I began to explore creating and living in a way that was reflected more balance between my masculine and feminine energy. As I begin to practice creating in a way that honoured my body, things began to feel completely different. Life felt way more spacious, more inspiring, and much more enjoyable.

HOW THE PROCESS OF CREATION LOOKS AND FEELS DIFFERENT WHEN WE EMBRACE OUR WHOLE BODY

When we create in an overly masculine way the process of creation feels completely different from what it does when we create in a more balanced way.

Creating in a masculine way *may* look like:

- Setting time frames, targets, and parameters
- Working to a schedule
- Creating from a results-driven approach
- Continuing even when we feel tired and exhausted
- Doing things the way they have always been done, because it works
- Playing by the rules

- Productivity is of utmost importance
- It's the outcome that matters, not the process

More importantly than what it looks like, is how creating in an overtly masculine way *may* feel:

- Full of effort and hard
- Restrictive
- Exhausting
- Like there is no time and space for rest, resetting, and recovery
- Like if you slow down, you will just stop
- Like we can rest and enjoy when it's done, but it never seems to get done
- Like we are always striving for an endpoint

Creating in a more balanced and feminine way, that embraces your body's natural rhythm *may* look like:

- Creating when inspiration hits, and resting when it starts to feel like a grind
- Spacious, with a deep appreciation for the process
- Allowing deep trust that the journey leads to an outcome, but without a fixation on what that outcome will be
- Creative, and open to new ways
- Moving with the ebb and flow

Again, creating with more balanced feminine energy *feels* totally different. It *may* feel:

- Light, spacious, joyful
- Like there is room to move

- When things feel effortful and hard, you can take a break knowing that this is not an optimal time for creation and that effort and energy is best spent elsewhere
- Curious and open, rather than rigid and conformed
- Moving with the energetic momentum, rather than pushing and forcing

THE BIRTH OF WOMB ENERGY AND THE OPENING OF THE PELVIC PORTAL

From my own personal experience, and from my experience working with new mothers, I have noticed that often, after childbirth, women are called back to their sacred centre, their womb space. Whether we realise it or not, as we grow and develop a baby in our womb, we spend time connecting with this space physically, emotionally, and energetically. During pregnancy we feel the sensations of a baby moving in our body, we connect with this space physically through touch as we tend to rub our lower abdomen more, and usually (though not always) we feel a loving connection with our baby

As we give birth, our pelvic floor and our cervix *opens and softens* to allow for the birth of our baby, and as this happens our uterus contracts strongly to help move the baby through the birth canal. It is this incredible opening and softening that we experience in our transition to motherhood on a physical and cellular level, as well as an energetic and spiritual level, that I believe opens a portal that is part of our initiation into motherhood. After birth, as our body continues to transition into new phases of life and as we grow into motherhood, our body uses this time of rest, recovery, restoration, and reflection to send us messages that connect us back to womb space. Those messages may be physical in nature, with the presence of deep core and pelvic floor changes, or more emotional and eso-teric, where we have a sense of being called into deeper purpose and meaning in our life. Birth is also the final transition phase wherein the spirit of our child has moved from the spiritual realm into the physical realm. I believe that with this transition phase, new levels of wisdom can be accessed by the mother, as she receives the energetic and physical gift that is her child.

This is a significant opportunity for women to come home to their body, to their centre, and to their womb space. I believe this happens *no matter how we give birth*. Though to experience the full power of this transition, we need to feel at peace with our birth, which is one reason why healing birth trauma is an important aspect for any woman wanting to sense the full power of her body and her womb. This opening of the pelvic portal and this new connection to our root - the root of who we are - is part of what I believe causes new mothers to go through a transition phase where we question every-thing and gain a new perspective on life.

After the birth of my first daughter, I felt consumed with a desire to lead a more creative, soul-driven life. Initially, I didn't even know that this was the desire that was calling me, let alone what that would look like for me. My transition into motherhood gifted me a new op-portunity for self-discovery. This sense of being called back strongly to womb space, to our truth, to our passion, to our desires, and a newfound sense of potential and possibility is what many new mothers talk about and experience. They may not have the words to articulate their experiences, but the sensation certainly exists. I sense that more women than not have this experience, but because our society doesn't support women in nurturing their intrinsic nature, and because many mothers don't feel supported in their transition to motherhood with the sacredness that we often yearn for, we don't have the language to understand what this overwhelming feeling is.

When we aren't practiced in listening to our body, we feel unsure of our body's language. We ignore it, without giving ourselves the time and spaciousness to listen to the subtle signals from our body.

The revelatory process that stems from the opening of the pelvic portal can be confronting, confusing, overwhelming, and exhausting. Particularly because we often move through it at the same time as we are nurturing the needs of babies and small children. The more we can soften and open to the process, as opposed to *trying* to get to a result, the more enjoyable the journey is. In essence, I believe we are being called back to being present in our journey of life, and the more we try to control and speed up the process to get to 'there' (wherever there is) the stronger and more challenging the lessons become.

THE BELLY

As already mentioned, the transverse abdominis (TA) has an important role within the deep core. When working in a normal motor pattern, the TA contracts and relaxes in synchronicity with the pelvic floor. The TA and pelvic floor are essentially a team of muscles that help to support our physical centre so that we have a strong foundation to move from. Many women tend to grip and hold the abdominal muscles, stemming from what we are taught good posture entails which is to stand up tall with our shoulders back and tummy in. Sometimes we have been taught by our coaches and trainers to "brace" or "engage" our core and sometimes it's because we don't like what our tummy looks like when it's relaxed.

Physically the TA does engage to create a solid base for us to move from, but like all muscles, it needs to have periods of relaxation as well as contraction. Often the TA muscles are bracing in overdrive, lacking periods of softness and relaxation. Energetically the

TA braces because we feel the need to defend and protect ourselves from being too "soft" or "sensitive". We build walls in our relationships and abdominal tension builds as though we are literally putting a wall up, not allowing room for fluidity and flexibility. We may feel like the world is doing things *to us* rather than *for us* and, instead of stepping into our personal power and taking radical responsibility for our actions and decisions, we try to place blame onto other people and give away our power. This leaves us feeling like our life looks a particular way because of something someone else did.

The energetic medicine that helps us to soften through the abdomen is allowing ourselves to soften in our lives. To strengthen through the abdomen, we need to create loving boundaries, live from our centre, speak our truth and step into our personal power.

If you notice that you hold tension in your abdomen, the following practices can help to invite softness within the abdomen.

- In a four-point kneeling position (on the hands and knees) allow the belly to hang. Notice how easy or challenging this is for you.
- As you breathe into the belly allow the belly to bulge and soften. Allow any tension to gently melt away. Imagine the sit bones softening away from one another, without bearing down on the pelvic floor muscles.
- In standing, place one hand beneath the navel to rest on the belly. Allow the belly to gently soften and bulge into your hand. Feel the pelvic floor soften, and the buttocks release.
- Lastly, use the 'belly springing' technique described in the Deep Core Connection Practice on p. 273 - 277.

THE BREATH

When I tune into the energy of the diaphragm, I sense the energy of the breath; the inhale of life force energy, the subtle pause between the inhale and the exhale, the energetic release that occurs with each exhale, and the clear ebb and flow of energy with the breath. There is such calm readily available to us, simply by tuning into the breath.

When we notice our breath - its pace, the length of each inhale and exhale, and what muscles are being used to generate our breath - we notice how our body reflects how we respond to our thoughts and feelings.

The difference between breathing slowly, with longer breaths that are generated by the diaphragm and belly, compared to fast, shallow breaths that are generated by the accessory muscles of our neck and shoulders is significant. When we become stressed and anxious, we breathe more like the latter. Tension in the neck, shoulders, and jaw starts to develop, which can ultimately result in pain and headaches. The feeling of being unable to take a deep breath that can accompany fast, shallow breathing can further heighten stress and anxiety.

When we notice how the muscles of our deep core respond to our breath in the Deep Core Connection Practice (p. 273 - 277) we can sense that the breath is the driver of the deep core energy system. The breath provides an access point for us to tune into our deep core energy and notice how our body is responding to our decisions, actions, and emotions. We can utilise this access point to notice when we are making choices that feel radically aligned to our truth and to who we are at our core, and when we moving in a direction that is not. The power and beauty of the breath is, not only does it reveal to us such a depth of information, it also helps us tune into the peace and calm that is readily available to us at any moment.

Anatomically the lungs hug the heart and physiologically they work in a powerful relationship together to pump blood and deliver oxygen throughout our body. Perhaps one of the easiest places to connect to our subtle body energy is in our heart space. We can sense joy, love, and happiness in our hearts as well as heartbreak and sadness. This connection is frequently talked about, well known, and appreciated. We can feel when our heart feels full and open. We can also sense when it feels closed down and shut off. When you sense how the lungs wrap around and hug the heart anatomically, and how the breath drives the movement of the pelvic floor and the belly, we begin to notice the intricate relationships of our core on a physical level. This same intricate relationship exists within the more subtle energy body.

SENSING WOMB AND PELVIC ENERGY

The energy within the pelvic bowl offers a strong reflection of how we are creating our life. In subtle energy medicine, the left side of the body represents the feminine energy and the right side of the body reflects the masculine energy. The feminine represents our 'being' energy, our willingness to nurture and live in accordance with our natural rhythm, to honour our body's cycles, and to rest, reset and restore. The masculine represents our 'doing' energy, our willingness to take action and to show up and share our truth. When we tune into the energy of our pelvic bowl, our ovaries, and uterus, we can sense how our body is responding to our process of creation.

From my work as a Pelvic Floor Physiotherapist, I can share with you what I have noticed regarding how women's bodies respond physically and energetically to how a woman is living and creating.

When women are living and creating in connection with their body, their pelvic bowl reflects that with a state of vitality, suppleness, strength, and tone. Physically, the muscles of the pelvic floor feel supple, and there is an evenness of tone on the left and right sides of the pelvic floor. During internal pelvic therapy women report an ability to sense a gentle pressure on the muscles of the pelvic floor without particular tension, pain, or decreased sensation. When meditating on the pelvic bowl, particularly on the energy of the ovaries and the womb space, women report a gentle warmth radiating evenly from the ovaries, and a sense of peacefulness within their womb space. They often describe a sensation of feeling at home, nourished, and nurtured when meditating on their womb and ovary energy.

When women are living and creating without the essential nourishment of the feminine, their pelvic bowl reflects this with a state of fatigue or exhaustion on the right side of the pelvic bowl, and a feeling of undernourishment on the left side of the pelvic bowl. Physically the muscles of the pelvic bowl often feel tight, tender, and sometimes painful on the right side of the pelvic floor. The left side of the pelvic floor muscles can be more difficult to activate and women often report less sensation (or an absence of sensation) on the left compared to the right.

When meditating on the pelvic bowl women often report a sensation of 'buzzing' and a scattered pulsating from the right ovary. They often use the words overworked and exhausted to describe how their right ovary feels. When meditating on the left ovary, women often share a sensation of numbness or absence, using the words 'shrivelled up', dark and cold to describe the energy here. When women have ignored or suppressed their feminine energy, meditating on their womb space can feel like coming home to their body and it can be peaceful, joyous, and relaxing. It's as though the womb space serves as a reminder of what life can feel like, and offers a sensation that our body is a safe place to be.

When women feel unsafe or uncomfortable being present within the pelvic bowl, there is generally one of two main descriptions. Either there is a global tension within the pelvic bowl that can cause pain and a stabbing sensation. In this instance, the body is shutting down and closing off this space to protect the inner being. For other women, a sensation of numbness is described, and they are able to articulate with a strong awareness that they leave their body and find it very difficult to stay present in this space. Meditating on the pelvic bowl, women often report difficulty connecting to the pelvic bowl as the ovaries and uterus often feel undernourished and difficult to sense. Women who experience these kinds of sensations respond well to a very gentle approach towards pelvic connection and nourishment, with a focus on feeling safe and in control. Rather than seeing this as an inability to tune into their womb space, I like to remind women that being able to sense this absence in sensation is, in fact, a connection in itself. This is the body's invitation to explore what this emptiness or numbness means for you. Questions like "How does this emptiness make me feel?", "What would provide energetic nourishment to me, and for this space in my body?", and "What is here that is asking to be expressed?" are helpful to explore this empty sensation further.

Women with symptoms of pelvic organ prolapse often report a sensation of feeling unsupported in their life, whether that be due to a difficulty in asking for support, or in receiving it.

Even though I have noticed these consistencies with the physical and energetic expression of the pelvic bowl, it's important to understand that your experience and what you sense in this part of your body will be unique to you. Women often have a blend of these patterns, and they can change periodically. What you feel in your body, and what you sense that means for you, is always reliable as long as you are being open and honest with yourself. You can't get your body's communication wrong as long as you are being kind and loving towards yourself and approaching this work with a very gentle curiosity. While I encourage you to use this information and insight to help guide your understanding of womb and pelvic bowl energy, I also urge you to trust what you sense and feel in your body. As you read your pelvic bowl energy, remember this is not designed to be an opportunity for you to judge or criticise yourself. As you bring the sensations of your body into your awareness, know that there is no right or wrong way to feel and that these sensations simply offer a way of communication.

The purpose of sensing and understanding your pelvic energy is to help you to know how to nourish yourself physically, energetically, and spiritually. The practices in this book are designed to help with both. These practices also help to detect what you may like to invite more of into your life, and what you may like to let go of. It's the integrated approach of learning how to read and nourish your pelvic and womb space, along with using your body's wisdom to help guide you, that makes this work so powerful. These practices are a way of working with your body using a gentle, safe, and self-led approach so that you can positively reconnect with your feminine body. Approaching these practices gently and in a way that feels safe is important. There is a big difference between stretching yourself and finding your edges of growth in a way that feels safe, versus pushing yourself to places that feel unsafe. The whole purpose of engaging in these practices is to feel secure, whole and at home in your body. Pushing to places that feel unsafe does not serve this intention and has the opposite effect. There are no milestones that need to be reached in any particular time frame with these practices. A kind and gentle approach will allow your journey to unfold in the perfect time for you.

PELVIC BOWL CONNECTION AND
AUTHENTIC VOICE EXPRESSION

There is a strong relationship between our pelvic bowl connection and authentic voice expression. When we are connected to the core of who we are, it makes sense that we are more able to speak in our authentic voice. Again, looking to the anatomical body and physiological relationship between the vocal cords and the pelvic floor helps to give more clarity and understanding of this energetic relationship.

Not only do the muscles of the vocal cords and the pelvic floor have similarities in their appearance, we also know that the breath is a driver for movement of the pelvic floor as well as the vocal cords. The pelvic floor softens and contracts in response to the breath, while the vocal cords rely on the breath to generate sound. At a primal level, women seem to innately know of the vocal cord and pelvic floor connection, naturally generating the low and deep guttural noises that promote pelvic floor softening and relaxation during childbirth and labour, and often expressing higher-pitched tones that promote pelvic floor tightening during sex.

PELVIC FLOOR & VOCAL CHORDS SIMILARITIES

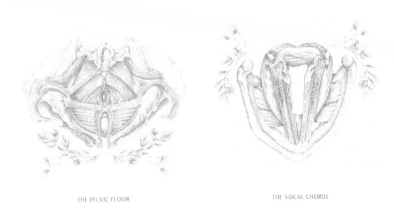

THE PELVIC FLOOR

THE VOCAL CHORDS

When we tune into our core energy, we can notice when our energy feels open, relaxed, and expansive, and when our energy feels contracted, closed off and restrictive. This information helps us to discern our truth, to express our truth, and give voice to our authentic self.

Many women that I work with who have pelvic pain and tightness (also known as pelvic hypervigilance or hypertonic pelvic floor or over activity of the pelvic floor), also have pain and tightness in their jaw, grind their teeth, and/or have concerns with regular throat infections or irritation. Over time, as we explore what is happening at an energetic level, it becomes clear to her that her pelvic tension and her tension around her throat is connected to not speaking her truth in some way.

These women often find creating deep humming sounds quite difficult. They share that it is difficult to perform physically and that they can sense their resistance to it. Practicing deep humming can help to relax the pelvic floor and it can also help to guide us towards the expression of our authentic voice by releasing built-up tension both within the vocal cords and the pelvis. Other breath practices such as deep sighing, extended pursed-lip exhalation through a soft jaw, and exhaling through a relaxed jaw to create lip vibration (also known as creating a motorboat sound) can also help to soften and relax both the jaw and pelvic floor.

Knowing what comes first, pelvic tension or difficulty with authentic voice expression can be a bit of a chicken or the egg situation. Often the two happen concurrently on some level, but one may be more prominent than the other. I believe to improve one we need to improve both - this is how interconnected the two are. Combining the Deep Core Connection Practice with deep humming is a nice place to start. Free-writing, or stream of consciousness writing (where you write whatever comes to your heart or mind and give it a place of expression) is also very helpful. Stream of consciousness writing can feel like your hand can't keep up with what's inside of you and that's OK. What you write doesn't need to be particularly legible or make any sense; it's the practice of expression that is important. An alternative is to record your voice in a voice memo on your phone. You may choose to go back and read or listen to what you have written, or if it feels like you have created space internally without the need to go back and reflect on what you have said/written then that is perfect too. Usually, I find it's getting it out of your mind/body and expressing it facilitates the healing that is desired. Burning or burying your paper with the intention to release it back to the Earth to absorb the energy and create something new and nourishing is a nice addition to this practice. Deleting a voice recording with acknowledgment of the newfound space within is just as powerful.

Although pelvic stress and jaw symptoms often occur concurrently, the correlation between authentic voice expression and pelvic symptoms is not limited to pelvic tension alone. The unexpressed energy can reveal itself in any form of core imbalance, pelvic stress, or silent pelvis symptoms. This is why creating space to reveal your true nature and full self is so important when treating pelvic symptoms. Managing the physical symptoms alone is essentially a Band-Aid approach where we ignore one of the major underlying causes of the symptoms.

Following are some questions for contemplation regarding creativity and authentic voice expression.

- How am I expressing myself creatively?
- How would I like to explore more creative expression?
- What holds me back from creative expression?
- If I was to explore my creative expression more fully, what would I do more of?
- Where in my life do I hold back in my self-expression?
- How do I feel about taking up space?
- If I trusted that what I have to offer the world is of value, how would I show up/share differently in my life?
- What would I like to do, but feel afraid to?
- If I knew I couldn't get it wrong, what would I be doing?
- If there were no boundaries and no limitations, what would I love to be doing?
- Where in my life am I being called to take action?
- What is the next best step?

COMMON PELVIC HEALTH CONCERNS

There are a number of common pelvic health concerns that women experience across the lifetime. Some of the most bothersome include prolapse, incontinence, and pelvic pain. In this section, I share more information regarding each of these conditions.

CORE IMBALANCE, PELVIC STRESS, AND SILENT PELVIS SYMPTOMS

What I term *core imbalance* other practitioners often refer to as "core dysfunction". Core imbalance is the term used to describe when the muscles of the core are not working in a well-coordinated fashion to create adequate core stability for a particular task. This may be due to a delayed contraction of a particular muscle/group of muscles, muscle overactivity, or lack of strength or endurance for particular tasks. Core imbalance can cause symptoms such as back pain, neck and shoulder pain, and many of the symptoms associated with pelvic stress.

When referring to collective pelvic floor symptoms, practitioners often use the term pelvic floor dysfunction. For a while, I did as well, until I realised how much meaning we can attach to this kind of terminology. To me, the term 'dysfunction' has a connotation that there is something wrong with the woman or her body. I prefer terms like *pelvic stress* or *silent pelvis* because they offer more of an understanding of what is happening at both an energetic and physical level, and also give hope that it is not necessarily the body's permanent state.

What I term *pelvic stress* is any pelvic symptom that is related to increased pelvic floor muscle tension *that creates undesirable side effects* including pelvic pain, pelvic organ prolapse (POP), incontinence, and painful sex. I believe the tension exists on both a physical and energetic level. It is surprising to many that POP and incontinence can be linked to a hypertonic or high tone pelvic floor because usually these symptoms are associated with a weak pelvic floor, which is not necessarily the case. I talk more about this in the section on incontinence and POP. What I consider to be a *silent pelvis* or *quiet pelvis* is one where the pelvic floor is less active on a muscular and/or energetic level.

From an energetic point of view, our core and pelvic energy can either feel open and expansive, restricted and contracted, or dull and muted. When our core or pelvic energy becomes restricted and contracted or dull and muted, we begin to feel the physical effects of this in the form of muscle tension or lack of muscular support respectively. Contracted core energy commonly expresses itself physically in the form of muscle tension in the pelvic region, neck, and shoulders, and jaw. Symptoms often include:

- Pelvic pain, including pain with sex
- Pelvic organ prolapse (POP) symptoms (see p. 120 - 121) and incontinence
- Neck and shoulder pain that can lead to headaches
- Jaw pain, a sometimes-dislocating jaw, and grinding teeth

Dull or muted energy is more likely to cause symptoms associated with decreased muscle tone in the pelvic region like prolapse, incontinence, and low back pain. Women with a silent/quiet pelvis often sense that their relationship with their feminine body has been suppressed and feel disconnected from their body. Common ways to describe the feeling within the silent pelvis are sad, tired, quiet, ignored, lonely, and unsupported.

PELVIC ORGAN PROLAPSE (POP)

As mentioned earlier, the pelvic floor is responsible for helping to support the pelvic organs (bladder, bowel, and uterus) and keep them in place. If the pelvic floor is unable to meet the demands placed upon it, POP can occur.

POP is the *symptomatic descent* of one or more of the anterior vaginal wall (that supports the bladder), the posterior vaginal wall (that supports the bowel), and the apex of the vagina (cervix/uterus) or vault after a hysterectomy (Abrams et al, 2017). Medical terminology referencing different kinds of POP exists and in the past, anterior wall prolapse was referred to as a cystocele, posterior wall prolapse was named a rectocele, and an apical prolapse was termed a uterine prolapse. New medical terminology requires a woman to have symptoms as well as increased movement of the vaginal walls for this diagnosis.

It is widely accepted that 50% of women will develop prolapse but only 10-20% of those seek evaluation for their condition. In the current literature, the overall prevalence of POP varies significantly depending upon the definition utilised, ranging from 3-50% (Abrams et al, 2017). In the past, only the descent of the organs was required for diagnosis and some health professionals will still use this older terminology. Interestingly, when POP is defined and graded on *symptoms*, the prevalence of it is 3-6% as compared to 41-50% when based on examination, as mild prolapse (Stage 1) on examinations is common and frequently asymptomatic (Abrams et al, 2017). According to recent research, it has become clear that Stage 1 anterior and posterior compartment descent is likely to be within normal range meaning that it is likely that POP has been over-diagnosed and that women who have been told they have a Stage 1 anterior or posterior wall prolapse are likely to have normal vaginal wall movement

(Buchsbaum et el., 2006; Dietz et el., 2016; Harmanli, 2014). I think this is important because often women are told they have a prolapse but experience no symptoms at all. In saying that, many women can feel quite disconnected from their feminine body and in some cases have reduced sensation in their pelvic and vaginal regions, meaning that they may not be aware of symptoms due to a physical and energetic dissociation from this space in their body.

The diagnosis of POP can be detrimental to the overall wellbeing of many women, particularly when they feel as though they need to change their lifestyle due to something that was causing them no concern at all. Often, the diagnosis of POP is delivered in very insensitive ways, with limited information about how it can be managed conservatively (without surgery) which adds to the stress and trauma of POP. When we are considering pelvic health in relation to POP, much care needs to be taken because it's important that women are well informed about prolapse so that they can make good lifestyle decisions when, at the same time, diagnosing prolapse can cause further disconnect and disassociation from the feminine body. This is why I believe a holistic and whole-body integrated approach to pelvic health serves women better than many of our existing models of care.

SYMPTOMS OF PELVIC ORGAN PROLAPSE

Following is a list of common symptoms women complain of associated with POP:

- A 'bulging' sensation in the vagina
- A heaviness or dragging sensation within the pelvis
- Lower back pain
- Difficulty initiating/completing a bladder/bowel motion

- Needing to support the vaginal walls to pass a bowel motion
- Incontinence or leakage from the bladder or the bowel
- A deep thudding sensation/pain with sex

HOW IS PELVIC ORGAN PROLAPSE DIAGNOSED?

The best way to receive an accurate diagnosis of pelvic organ prolapse is to have an *internal vaginal pelvic floor assessment by a pelvic floor physiotherapist.*

During this assessment your therapist should be able to assess and tell you about:

- The strength, endurance, and coordination of your pelvic floor muscles
- The degree of descent of the anterior (front) and posterior (back) vaginal walls and cervix
- Objective measurements that help to inform you of the likelihood of developing vaginal wall descent

THINGS TO KNOW ABOUT PROLAPSE DIAGNOSIS

It can change!

Certainly, what a pelvic floor therapist observes during an assessment on one particular day may be different from another. There can be multiple reasons for this, including:

- The time of day you were seen - generally later in the day, as gravity has had more effect, prolapse makers are more noticeable.
- The amount of movement and exercise you have done, for the same reasons mentioned above.

- How far along in your postnatal journey you are if you have had a baby - in the very early postnatal phases after a vaginal delivery, increased movement of the vaginal walls can be expected. There will be some natural improvement as the body heals.
- Where you are in your cycle – as mentioned in the 'Menstrual Magic' section of this book, where you are in your menstrual cycle can have an effect on prolapse and POP symptoms.

Get checked in the position you have symptoms in

If you have symptoms of pelvic organ prolapse, I recommend you ask your chosen therapist to assess your pelvic floor in the position where you are most aware of your symptoms. What can be observed in a supine (lying position) will be different from what can be observed in a standing position. It's becoming more common practice for therapists to offer pelvic checks in a standing position, but some therapists may practice this less than others.

You have a choice!

It seems so obvious to say that when it comes to the treatment and management of POP, you have a choice! Unfortunately though, like many things pertaining to women's health, we have treatments thrust upon us, sometimes without all available options being presented to us, and often with many assumptions being made. If you choose, you can do nothing at all. You have the right to informed choice, which means being given all of your treatment options along with their likelihood of success and failure, and any potential side effects.

You have the right to feel informed, respected, supported, valued, and heard. When you are being presented with treatment options, it should feel like a conversation where you get to ask questions and share your thoughts and feelings. It shouldn't feel like you are being told what to do. Your body, your choice. Simple.

Your diagnosis does not define you

Here I am specifically referring to the diagnosis of POP, but I do believe that this same conversation can be relevant for many of the diagnoses we can be given. Your diagnosis does not define you.

It saddens me that I've met so many women who've been diagnosed with POP with no symptoms to complain of, during a passing comment with no consideration given to the impact that this would have on the woman and her life. Often upon assessment what I observe is what is clinically considered normal vaginal wall movement, sometimes slightly increased vaginal wall movement that's synonymous with having given birth. I would argue that the diagnosis itself is inaccurate. More importantly, it's the lack of conversation that takes place after this diagnosis has been given, with women being left feeling completely alone and wondering what the presence of POP may mean for her as an individual. Often, the little discussion that does occur consists of the health professional dictating to the woman what she is allowed to and not allowed to do with her body and what her life will look like now that she knows she has a prolapse.

The problem is that when a health professional (or anyone for that matter) tells a woman what she can and can't do with her body, that professional often has very little understanding of what any of these now forbidden activities (like running) actually mean to that woman. Telling them what they should and shouldn't be doing and making them feel wrong if they choose otherwise isn't kind, nor is it helpful.

Sure, informed choice is important and health professionals are experts in their own right. Their role is to provide evidence-based information and offer guidance. However, when the choice is taken away, it's no longer an informed decision. It's a brutal disempowerment.

HOW IS PELVIC ORGAN PROLAPSE
MANAGED / TREATED?

There is a range of treatment options for pelvic organ prolapse. As mentioned earlier, it's important to know that there is both a muscular and fascial component to the pelvic floor and that both the muscles and the fascia provide support to the pelvic organs. When it comes to the muscular component we can strengthen and condition the pelvic floor with exercise, massage, breathwork, motor re-patterning techniques, and relaxation exercises. Some ligamentous and connective tissue changes are not reversible, and therefore don't respond particularly well to manual therapy or exercise therapy, which means some kind of additional support may be required. The muscular system offers additional support to the fascial components of the pelvic floor, which is why healthy pelvic floor muscles are important.

It is a common misconception that a lack of strength is the only cause of pelvic floor symptoms. While that is sometimes the case, it's not always. When the muscles of the pelvic floor are too tense, or in 'overdrive', they lack the relaxation that is required for healthy muscle function. If you imagine clenching your fist all day, the muscles of your hand would fatigue prematurely, and this clenched position doesn't offer optimal hand functioning. This is the same within the pelvis. When the muscles of the pelvic floor are clenching tightly and lack softness, they maintain a state of contraction. Rather than being able to lift and provide additional support in response to certain movement patterns, the muscles of the pelvic floor have nowhere to go. Imagine tightening your biceps muscle as firmly as possible and then asking your muscles to contract further to lift something. It's impossible. It is in this way that a hypertonic pelvic floor can contribute to ongoing pelvic symptoms, including pelvic pain and symptoms of pelvic organ prolapse. You can see how the assumption that weakness is always the concern is unhelpful. This is why it's helpful to have the guidance of a pelvic floor therapist who can tell you more about your pelvic health.

Pelvic floor physiotherapists grade pelvic floor muscle strength on a scale from 0-5:

- 0 = no muscle activity able to be detected
- 1 = a flicker of muscle activity able to be felt
- 2 = muscle activity felt, but through a small range of motion only
- 3 = muscle activity felt through the full range of motion against gravity without additional resistance
- 4 = muscle activity through the full range of movement with resistance
- 5 = muscle activity through the full range of movement against maximal resistance

When it comes to pelvic floor strength, not all women require grade 5 strength. What is required is an adequate level of strength to help support our pelvic organs during our day-to-day tasks. The amount of strength that one woman requires may be completely different from another because their lifestyle and physical activity levels will be different. A CrossFitter who works as a nurse, for example, will require more strength than someone who prefers swimming and works in an office.

Pelvic floor exercises can help to strengthen and condition the pelvic floor, and therefore create additional support for the pelvic organs. There are several ways that you can help to strengthen, improve coordination, and increase the endurance of the pelvic floor – I talk about this more in additional sections of this book.

LIFESTYLE MODIFICATIONS:

Lifestyle modification is another option in helping to treat pelvic organ prolapse (POP). You may be aware of specific activities that aggravate your POP symptoms. Lifestyle modification requires us to change some aspect of these activities, whether that means reducing their intensity or duration, or perhaps stopping the activity altogether. If you're considering these changes as part of POP management, it's important to consider how meaningful particular activities are to you. Ceasing certain things that we love and enjoy may be more detrimental to our health than the POP itself, meaning the treatment causes more issues than the problem itself. If you do choose lifestyle modification as part of your management plan, know that this doesn't always mean stopping a particular activity. There are many ways that we can modify our movement, and it might be that a simple tweak is all that is required to improve your symptoms rather than ceasing the activity altogether. Lastly, know that your lifestyle modifications don't need to be forever. Perhaps you make some changes while your body recovers (in the postnatal period, for example) or while you strengthen and condition the muscles of the pelvic floor. It may also be that you only need to modify these activities during particular phases of your cycle, for example in the days leading up to your period and the days of your period.

PESSARIES:

Pessaries are silicone-based supports designed to help support the vaginal walls and give additional lift to the pelvic organs. There are many different kinds of pessaries, but the most common are the ring pessary and the cube pessary.

One of the major differences between the two is that a ring pessary can remain inserted in the vagina for longer periods (up to 12 months), which means they can also be worn during intercourse, and women can use tampons at the same time. Due to the placement of a ring pessary, they also tend not to interrupt menstrual blood flow but because they sit quite high within the vagina and don't have a string to help remove them, they can be more challenging for women to remove themselves. This is another reason why we tend to recommend that they stay in place for longer periods, and are taken out and changed/renewed by a pelvic floor therapist.

Cube pessaries, on the other hand, are designed to be inserted for use during the daytime or for a particular activity (such as exercise) then removed. Cube pessaries have a string attached, which means that women can insert and remove them with ease. Cube pessaries cannot be worn during intercourse or at the same time as tampons. Cubes do somewhat interrupt menstrual blood flow, though not entirely, which is sometimes not desirable for women who like to sense a free-flow.

Pessaries can be fitted by trained pelvic floor physiotherapists and monitored with shared care by your pelvic floor physio and your GP. They are an alternative to surgery, offer much fewer risks to women, and have a high level of success. (Abdol et al, 2011; De Albuquerque Coelho et al, 2016; Dumoulin et al 2018; Handa and Jones, 2002) Pessaries don't come without risk but generally, when cared for well, they have very few side effects. Often women aren't offered the chance to trial pessaries despite the evidence supporting them and low risk. This is perhaps because often when women are diagnosed with POP they are referred to gynaecologists who tend to offer surgery because surgery is what they know and are trained in.

There are multiple reasons I think pessaries are a good option for women to consider:

- You can trial them to see if you like them, and stop using them if they don't. This is not the case with surgery.
- They have fewer risks than surgery and often have the same or better results.
- They are cost-effective.
- They can also provide peace of mind and feedback during exercise and activity (more on that next).
- You have autonomy of how and when to use a pessary. You can choose to use them when required, and take them out when you don't feel the need for them.

Even though well-fitted pessaries are unable to be felt once inserted, some women don't like the thought of pessaries for different reasons, often because they don't like the thought of it being inserted into their vagina. If you do choose to use a pessary, you don't need to use it all of the time. Some women use them for the purpose of exercise alone. Some women only use them when they have symptoms. Some women use them just for the week leading up to their period when they know that they experience more heaviness.

HOW PESSARIES CAN BE USED FOR PEACE OF MIND AND FEEDBACK DURING EXERCISE

There is a certain population of women who may like to use a pessary for peace of mind and to offer feedback during exercise. I am one of them! Some women who have an increased risk of prolapse, or have some degree of prolapse, may choose to use a support pessary during higher impact and higher intensity exercise like running and weightlifting. Even if they have adequate strength, endurance and coordination to maintain adequate pelvic support during exercise, it can give some women peace of mind to use a pessary so that they can feel more confident and comfortable during activity and movement. By taking notice of any migration or downward movement of the pessary during and after exercise, either by sensing the shift vaginally or by inserting a finger into the vagina to see if it has changed position at all, pessaries can also act as a feedback mechanism. Using pessaries in this way is becoming more common as women continue with high-intensity exercise such as running and CrossFit after having children, and as we understand more about the potential impact of high intensity of exercise in relation to POP. In my opinion, this is an option for women to consider, and to use if it feels right for them. For me personally, it gave me peace of mind to continue with exercise that I loved and enjoyed and to gain confidence in my body after birth. I wish to be clear, though, that this is *not* a way to try and 'fast forward' any recovery or rebuilding after birth. It may also not feel like a good option for you, and that is perfectly fine too. The important thing for me is that we are offered a choice.

SURGERY

To be honest, I only want to touch briefly on surgery as a treatment option for POP. Surgery has high risks associated with it, and often low success rates. In one particular study, 35.4% of women reported return of symptoms within three (3) months of POP surgery and the median duration for return of symptoms was 6 months. (Johnson et al, 2013). The devastating effects of surgical mesh used in prolapse surgery have led to an international inquiry regarding the efficacy of certain surgical interventions for prolapse. Whilst I acknowledge that surgery is a valuable option for some women, this is not an area of expertise that I feel qualified to dive deeply into. If you are considering surgery, I urge you to make sure you are well informed of both. It's also important to consider how the surgery may change your life. Do you anticipate that it will have a significantly positive impact? Or is it likely that your activities would look much the same, or become more limited? Weighing up the impact of the prolapse and how it affects your day-to-day against the potential impacts of surgery is an important part of the process of considering if surgery is right for you. If you experience minimal to no POP symptoms, how will undergoing surgery make your life look and feel different? These are just some of the questions to consider when making your decision. Some surgeons will also offer additional surgical intervention concurrent to POP surgery, such as Hysterectomy. It's important to know why any surgery would be indicated. It is important to consider questions like: What are the likely benefits? What risks are involved? How may surgical intervention likely change your overall outcome? Simply having a Hysterectomy because you have finished having children, for example, may not be a strong enough reason to consent to a Hysterectomy.

INCONTINENCE (BLADDER AND BOWEL)

Incontinence is unwanted leakage from the bladder or the bowel. There are two main types of urinary incontinence, urge urinary incontinence (UUI) and stress urinary incontinence (SUI).

SUI affects about 1 in 3 women after birth, and although it is common it isn't something to be ignored. Unfortunately, because leakage is common, it's often accepted as normal. Pad and sustainable underwear companies often use language that further nor-

| 130 |

malises incontinence like, "Everybody leaks sometimes!" and suggest that the solution is to simply use their product. While these products play an important role in helping women feel secure in their body, it's the normalisation of incontinence, along with only offering a Band-Aid solution that sometimes has women feeling that they have to live with this, rather than knowing that they can do something about it. As the collective voice of women's health practitioners becomes louder, and particularly that of women's pelvic health therapists, more women are recognising that there is help available to them. Women don't need to laugh it off or put up with this very confronting and often debilitating concern. There is strong evidence to show that supervised pelvic floor exercise can help to improve or fully resolve bladder incontinence (Dumoulin et al, 2018). Although not supervised, the exercises in this book are the same exercises that you would be participating in during a supervised program.

Stress Urinary Incontinence (SUI) is the involuntary leakage of urine on effort or physical exertion, and times that increase intra-abdominal pressure. (i.e. physical stress on the bladder) Common examples of increased intra-abdominal pressure/exertion include coughing, laughing, sneezing, lifting heavy weight/s, and jumping. SUI occurs because urethral pressure (which keeps the urethra closed) cannot be maintained high enough during times of increased intra-abdominal pressure (IAP). There are several causes of insufficient urethral pressure:

- Poorly coordinated bracing of the pelvic floor during times of increased IAP in which learning 'The Knack' (p. 150 - 151) and practicing pelvic floor coordination exercises will be helpful

- A weakness of the muscles of the pelvic floor, in which pelvic floor strength training is beneficial
- Damage to the pelvic fascia, in which case a support pessary or tampon may be useful
- Inner urethral factors such as loss of urethral sphincter muscle fibres, and decreased oestrogen, in which case pelvic floor muscle training can be helpful (as the same nerve that innervates the pelvic floor innervates the urethral sphincter) or oestrogen therapy may be beneficial

Urge urinary incontinence (UUI) is leakage accompanied or immediately preceded by urgency. Urgency is a sudden and intense desire to void. Urgency is a complex mechanism and is likely to have different underlying causes in different women. Common triggers for urgency can be the sound of running water, seeing a toilet, and sometimes putting a key in the door (knowing that the toilet is on the other side). The pelvic floor should be able to override these triggers, but in the case of urge incontinence, it can't. Treating UUI requires us to dissociate from these triggers using distraction techniques as well as our body's neural pathways. During times of urgency, women have a strong instinctive urge to race to the toilet. The problem with doing this is that at these times is that if you suddenly begin racing to the toilet, you add even greater pressure to your bladder increasing the chance you will experience leakage of urine.

Behaviour retraining is about changing how you react to these intense episodes of urgency. The first step is to realise that if you can wait a minute or by using the following techniques, the urgency will often pass. Waiting and walking (rather than running) to the toilet after the urgency has passed will mean you are less likely to leak.

Here are some techniques that help relax the bladder during episodes of urgency:

- Counting backward from 100 by 7's
- Applying pressure with the fingers on the perineum (the space between the vagina and anus) OR to be more discreet you can sit on your heel
- Standing on tippy toes or doing calf raises
- Curling your toes
- Stopping and breathing slowly, deeply, and calmly

Faecal urgency (FU) and faecal incontinence (FI) is less common than UI but is certainly a disturbing concern for women. Faecal incontinence is far less talked about than UUI, SUI, and POP, and few women (less than 10%) seek help for their symptoms. Women who experience FI have usually experienced a larger perineal tear, known as obstetric anal sphincter injuries or OASIS. Third and fourth-degree perineal tears are the primary risk factor for FI and it is more prevalent if forceps were used to assist the delivery of a baby (Johannessen et al 2014). FI is also associated with a dramatic increase of dyspareunia (pain with sex) at 3-6 months post-birth. If you have experienced a perineal tear, you may or may not know to what degree. If you do experience FI, finding out what degree of tear you had and how it was managed can be important information to help you if you choose to seek help. Know that you can request this information from your care provider and that this information must be made accessible to you. It is not reasonable to be denied access to this information, and if you are it is important to know that in Australia you have a right to be granted access to your personal health information and records from any person who provides health care to you.

Because of the lower incidence of FI, as well as the fact that far fewer women seek help for their symptoms, there are fewer pelvic floor physiotherapists whose expertise is in FI. However, this doesn't mean that help does not exist. To seek help for FI requires deep self-compassion, courage, and being gentle with yourself in your approach to any type of therapy. Remember that the physical symptoms are just one aspect of FI and having space to safely voice your emotions and experiences may be very helpful. Living in silence makes us feel further alone and isolated. You are not alone, and help is available.

LEAKAGE AFTER SWIMMING, BATHING OR PERIODS OF WATER IMMERSION

Often postnatal women experience what they refer to as leakage after periods of water immersion, whether that be swimming or bathing. This type of leakage is different from stress or urgency incontinence because it is *only* experienced after water immersion, and feels like water that has entered the vagina is leaking out, rather than it being urine. Similar to the cause of vaginal flatus, this leaking relates to water entering the space in the vagina. After being immersed in the water, it is on returning to land that the water leakage can be felt.

There is limited evidence on water immersion leakage and the best treatment for this. If you find it particularly bothersome you may like to trial some kind of space-occupying device such as a Contiform/board pessary, a cube pessary, or a tampon. For most women, knowing the cause of the leakage and understanding that it is different from urinary incontinence gives them good peace of mind.

HEALTHY BLADDER HABITS

Normal voiding frequency is suggested as voiding 4-6 times per day or voiding every 3-4 hours, keeping in mind that the amount of fluid you consume, as well as how much you sweat will have an impact on this. The impact of bladder concerns such as urgency (a sudden intense desire to void), frequency (increased number of times urinating during the day), and incontinence (leakage from the bladder) have significant impacts on our quality of life that surpass physical concerns alone. In one particular study, two-thirds of the 206 women in the study were worried about having a bad odour and felt that they were less attractive, 50% were anxious that others would discover their 'problem' and 38% of men (partners to patients) reported that the bladder concerns harmed their relationship. (Nilsson et al, 2009)

In another study, it was found that the impact of similar bladder concerns had a major impact on the individual and family members. Urinary frequency impacted both the woman and her family in the way of travel, social activities, sleep, sex, and intimacy, along with the emotional impacts of worry, embarrassment, anger, and frustration. (Coyne et al, 2009)

Maintaining healthy bladder habits can help to prevent bladder conditions from occurring, and can help to resolve already existing bladder problems. Healthy bladder habits include:

Avoiding going to the toilet 'just in case'.

Going 'just in case' can reduce the bladder's capacity to stretch. This reduced stretch happens both on a physical level and a neurological level, meaning that the reduced stretch can cause increased bladder sensation and increased urinary frequency. Ultimately this can lead to a further decrease in bladder compliance, and the spiral continues. Decreased bladder compliance can lead to increased urinary frequency, which can ultimately lead to urgency and urge in-continence.

When you sense the need to urinate, *don't answer the "first call"-wait 10 minutes*. Again, this relates to maintaining bladder compliance and healthy bladder functioning at a neurological and physical level.

Maintaining your hydration.

This is important for general health, and the health of the bladder itself. Acidic urine can lead to increased urinary frequency, and ultimately lead to urinary urgency and urge incontinence. Although there is much education around drinking a particular amount of fluid each day, the best way to monitor your hydration is to look at the colour of your urine. This is because we all live in different environments, sweat differently, and use our bodies differently. Someone doing little movement, in a cool environment, who is not sweating at all will need less fluid to maintain their hydration compared to a woman who is going for a run in the heat of the day.

Adequate hydration is reflected by urine that is pale and straw-like in colour, anything darker indicates the need to drink more fluids. If your urine is almost clear, you may opt to drink a little less particularly if you are finding frequency a concern. Don't take too much notice of the colour of your urine the very first time you go to the bathroom in the morning as your kidneys have been working overnight without much fluid input and will therefore naturally produce darker coloured urine.

Notice also the flow of urine.

The flow of urine should be easy to commence, with a steady stream, and stop completely without dribbling or the sensation of needing to go again shortly after. There are many reasons why the flow of urine may become disrupted including pelvic organ prolapse (POP), a bladder outlet obstruction, or decreased bladder muscle activity. Knowing the cause of an altered flow of urine can help to manage the primary problem early and prevent further conditions from developing such as urinary tract infections (UTIs), or the progression of POP.

Lastly, it's important *not to ignore symptoms such as bladder leakage and urgency.* Symptoms of increased urinary urgency or incontinence may be a result of an underlying concern that may require further investigation or intervention. In addition, these symptoms can be the precursor to secondary conditions and without appropriate management it is increasingly likely that they will develop.

HEALTHY BOWEL HABITS

Maintaining healthy bowel habits helps to maintain our overall health and to prevent possible pelvic floor concerns from developing. One of the major muscles of the pelvic floor, the puborectalis muscle, forms a sling that originates from the pubic bone and wraps around the rectum and back to the pubic bone. The puborectalis muscle creates a 'kink' in the rectum and helps to maintain faecal continence. When we sit well on the toilet this muscle can relax to unkink the bowel and help stools to pass freely through the rectum. When we don't sit well on the toilet, or when we are constipated, we need to generate more force through the pelvic floor to pass bowel motions. When this occurs there is increased downward pressure onto the pelvic floor that can increase the risk of developing POP.

The main things to note concerning toilet posture are:

- Sit with the knees higher than the hips, preferably by using some kind of stool/foot support. The neural pathways that help us to press up onto our toes are the same as those that help to maintain continence. Think about young children who dance on their tip-toes when they need to use the bathroom – this is one of our body's natural ways to stop us from leaking. This is why a stool is preferred so that we don't have to work against this natural neural pathway.

- Have the knees slightly wider than the hips to allow for a gentle lean forward from the hip joint and an open outlet.
- Keep the back relatively straight to avoid compression on the abdomen.
- Allow the belly to soften and bulge.
- Don't push, simply allow the bowel motion to fall away naturally.

Bringing awareness to your bowel motions is the best way to monitor your bowel health. The Bristol Stool Chart indicates what a healthy bowel motion looks like. A copy of the Bristol Stool Chart is readily available on the internet through a simple Google search.

A stool Type 3 or 4 is considered ideal for optimal bowel and pelvic health. Bowel motions should be soft and easily passed without the need to strain. If you do experience constipation, increasing green leafy vegetable intake, fruit content, as well as fluid in your diet may be helpful. If you choose to use natural fibre supplements or other stool softeners, be aware that some bulking agents can help stool consistency long-term but they can cause worsening constipation of you are already constipated. Ideally, constipation should first be addressed with an appropriate laxative medication (speak with your health care provider) and then the bulking agent used as a preventative measure for long-term prevention of constipation. Regular exercise can also help with bowel motility.

Unlike the bladder, it is encouraged that you answer the 'first call' of the bowel whenever possible.

In addition to healthy bladder and bowel habits, there are some other general health habits that can help to maintain pelvic health.

- Listening to your body during exercise, *and not ignoring symptoms of POP or incontinence* is important for pelvic health. You will find more detail on this in the sections that cover POP and incontinence.
- *Maintaining a healthy weight* is essential to pelvic health. Excessive weight puts additional pressure onto the pelvic floor.
- Coughing and sneezing create a tremendous load for the muscles of the pelvic floor so *managing chronic cough or sneezing* will reduce the load on the pelvic floor and therefore helps with overall pelvic health.
- Finally, learning *'The Knack' (p. 150 - 151)* and *exercising and/ or relaxing the pelvic floor* is recommended for women who have pelvic concerns.

PELVIC PAIN

Pelvic pain is a global term used for a range of conditions that cause pain within the pelvis including endometriosis, primary dysmenorrhea, and dyspareunia. Pelvic pain conditions are prevalent and have a huge impact on girls, women, and their families.
Endometriosis:

- 1 in 10 girls experience pelvic pain that severely impacts their schooling, career path, social growth, and participation.
- 1 in 10 women suffer from endometriosis.
- 1 in 3 women with endometriosis experience fertility problems.

- Seven to 12 years is the average delay between onset and diagnosis.
- Endometriosis is often associated with decreased social and economic participation, co-morbidities, and progression to chronic pelvic pain.
- Women and girls who have close relatives with endometriosis are 7-10 times more likely to develop it.
  (Australia. Australian Government Department of Health, 2018).

Dysmenorrhea:

- Primary dysmenorrhea is menstrual pain without identifiable organic cause, whereas a diagnosis of secondary dysmenorrhoea means there is an identifiable cause for the menstrual pain.

Evidence regarding exercise and physiotherapy treatments for women who experience pelvic pain for a whole range of reasons is continuing to evolve. In my experience of working with women who have pelvic pain a whole-body integrated approach that supports the woman holistically is most effective. Some women with high tone or hypertonic pelvic floor muscles experience generalised pelvic pain. Increased pelvic tone may be a result of a primary condition such as endometriosis, or it may be a standalone concern. Women with increased pelvic tone often experience tightness of the hips, inner thighs, glutes and abdominals. Down training of the muscles through muscle relaxation techniques such as stretching, massage and focused deep breathing can be helpful. Body awareness practices such as the Body Scan Practice (see page 271 - 273) are also beneficial.

VAGINAL FLATUS

Evidence suggests that the mechanism of vaginal wind (sometimes called queefing) may be due to the creation of a "valve-like structure at the entrance of the vagina, together with a real, rather than potential vaginal space". (Krissi et al, 2003)

Most women describe experiencing vaginal flatus during exercise that involves inverted manoeuvres like Pilates and yoga. Typically women can feel the air entering the vagina during the inversion, and then notice (and usually hear) its release when they return to an upright position. This can be embarrassing and distressing for women, particularly for those who enjoy practicing in a group setting.

From the very little evidence available to us, it is suggested that vaginal wind does not appear to be related to pelvic floor muscle weakness and does not appear to respond to pelvic floor muscle exercises. There is, however, anecdotal evidence that some women do respond to using 'The Knack' (page 150 - 151) prior to and during inverted moves. There is also a school of thought that says if we can increase our vaginal muscle bulk, then this real, rather than potential, space can be decreased. Evidence does show that vaginal wind does appear to be related to pelvic organ prolapse (POP) but it can occur in the absence of POP. Vaginal wind appears most successfully treated by a vaginal support/space-occupying devices such as a Contiform/Board Pessary, a cube pessary, or a tampon. (Franco and Fines, 2008; Krissi et al, 2003; Sylvia, 2007)

PELVIC CARE

This section will discuss physiotherapy techniques and lifestyle choices that you can integrate into your whole body health approach to pelvic care. Using these techniques alongside the Body Connection Practices in this book in a way that resonates with you is what creates an integrated approach towards pelvic health.

FINDING A PELVIC HEALTH THERAPIST

Being such an intimate part of our body, we need to choose our pelvic health practitioners with care. Finding someone that helps you feel seen, heard, and valued is important. Here are some things you may like to consider when choosing your pelvic health professional.

- Take a look at their website, their social media, and their marketing. Do they use language that resonates with you?
- Ask about their appointment lengths – do you feel like you will have enough time to feel seen and heard without feeling rushed?
- Do you sense that they have an open mind to working with you as a unique individual, or do you sense otherwise?
- Let your intuition guide you.
- If you do happen to work with a therapist that doesn't feel right, know that you can always choose another.

PELVIC EXAM ANXIETY

The thought of a pelvic exam can be quite unnerving for many women. There are many reasons why women will avoid a pelvic exam, and I want to help put your mind at ease.

Here are a few common reasons why women avoid pelvic exams:
Feeling afraid of knowing what the problem is.

Often when I assess and treat women, they are so surprised that their pelvic health is better than they anticipated. Sometimes what we imagine our pelvic health to be is far more catastrophic than re-ality. Knowing where you are at, and what you can do to help treat and manage any pelvic health concerns can be deeply empowering. It can also put your mind at ease from the scenarios you are making up in your head.

Thinking your vulva looks strange.

Trust me when I say this: the anatomy of your vulva doesn't look strange. I've seen hundreds of vaginas and none of them look the same. Sure, there are similarities but we are all different. Don't be fooled by what you see on TV, in magazines, or even in anatomy textbooks –women's bodies are modified in the media to look like a particular stereotype that simply doesn't reflect the majority of the population.

Feeling concerned you haven't 'groomed' yourself in a while.

Pubic hair is beneficial to maintaining vaginal health. Whether you choose to wax, shave, laser, or do no grooming at all is your per-sonal choice. Even if you do usually remove/trim your public hair and haven't in a while, your health care provider will think nothing of it. Never apologise for how you choose for your pubic hair to be, or how it happens to be at the time of an appointment.

Being worried you might leak.

If you were to leak during your assessment, you would certainly NOT be the only woman who has experienced that. Therapists an-ticipate that it is possible that you may leak during a pelvic exam.

Feeling like you don't know enough about your female body and are worried that you will appear unintelligent.

In my experience, many women feel so grateful to learn about their female anatomy and are quite surprised by how little they knew about their own bodies. Getting to know your feminine body helps you to gain more autonomy in monitoring and maintaining your pelvic health. There is no expectation or prerequisite knowledge!

This is not a test. Knowing your body will also help you to teach the important girls and women in your life about their health, which is all part of the powerful ripple effect that you can have in creating change around women's health.

You have financial concerns. What if you start a treatment you can't continue to afford?

Pelvic health therapy is an investment. Like anything, it can appear expensive, or it can be seen as highly valuable depending on your priorities, your personal experience, and your values. Ultimately you are in charge of how much you are willing to invest in your pelvic health. You don't need to feel pressured into continuing with treatments that are causing financial stress or strain. Finding a therapist that respects your autonomy, your resources, your values, and how you want to invest in your pelvic health is important. Reading my tips on finding the right therapist for you may be helpful.

You're not even sure that it's the right type of therapy for you.

Sometimes women are very clear on why they are coming to see me. For example, they have recently had a baby and want to review their pelvic health, understand the condition of their pelvic floor, and know how to move forward safely, smartly, and strongly. Other times, women who choose to work with me feel unsure of why exactly they have been drawn to the type of work that I do. They say that they didn't know what to expect, but deep within they just knew that this was their next right step. They were open, curious, and followed the breadcrumbs. This is exactly what using your body wisdom is about, following that intuition and guidance, even when it doesn't seem to make complete sense.

Usually, when a woman sees a pelvic health therapist who is a good fit for her, she will walk away with a better understanding of herself and her pelvic health, which is a win. If you do seek pelvic floor therapy and find that you only needed a one-off therapy/treatment that then helped you to continue on your pathway, it has served you perfectly.

You're concerned it might be painful.

Pelvic assessments should never be painful. For women who experience pain with penetration, the concern that a pelvic exam may be painful is very understandable. Good pelvic health professionals will allow you to be in control of the assessment and treatment every step of the way. Some women do worry if they are unable to have a complete exam, that they are wasting their time and their health care provider's time. This is not the case at all. A pelvic assessment is always complete, even when the reason for stopping is patient/client discomfort – whether that is physical or emotional. That in itself is all the information that is required to proceed with treatment and care advice. You never need to push through any pain with pelvic health therapy.

You've experienced previous pelvic trauma.

This is perhaps the biggest and least talked about concern that women have in relation to pelvic exams. Whether previous trauma is related to sexual assault, birth trauma, or medical trauma, it has a physical, emotional, and psychological impact that can lead to a sense of uneasiness when approaching pelvic assessments. Knowing that you can be totally in control of how a pelvic assessment goes can be the assurance that you need to feel comfortable and confident about a pelvic health assessment. In my experience, when I ask women, "What do you need to make this feel safe and comfortable for you?" they will generally know what that is. Sometimes the woman would like reassurance that if she is unable to continue with the pelvic assessment or treatment for any reason, that the therapist/professional won't feel offended, or like the woman has 'wasted their time'. Some women want to experience the touch of the practitioner to a different part of their body first. For other women, being in control and guiding the assessment themselves is powerful. In this case, I ask the woman to let me know when to start the assessment/treatment, when to progress and when to stop. For example, the woman tells me when she is going to perform a pelvic floor contraction, rather than me cueing her to perform the contraction.

Not all therapists will ask what it is that you sense will make you feel safe and comfortable but posing this question to yourself before a pelvic exam will help *you* to know what it is you need to feel safe and comfortable to proceed with an assessment or treatment. Tell your practitioner what you need to feel safe. If they are unwilling to hear that, they are not the right therapist for you.

If we consider the consistent message that 'women's bodies are wrong', messages that breed shame, guilt, doubt, and poor body image - it's no wonder that women feel anxious and uneasy at the thought of pelvic exams. The reclamation of the pelvic space through kind, gentle, and loving spaces where women feel held, safe, and comfortable helps to heal this long-learned pattern of pelvic shame that crosses generations.

EXERCISING THE PELVIC FLOOR

When it comes to pelvic health, most women are aiming for adequate pelvic floor function, which means having the strength, endurance, and coordination that is required to ensure that they do not experience pelvic symptoms such as prolapse or incontinence. Strength helps to generate enough force to maintain continence and pelvic organ support during activity, coordination helps the muscles to contract fast enough to maintain continence during a cough for example (sometimes it's not that the muscles are weak but just slow to contract - which means the cough is over before they got a chance to contract) and sufficient endurance is required to get us to the end of the day, or the end of a run.

PELVIC FLOOR STRENGTH

As already mentioned, not all women require 5/5 strength of the pelvic floor. Just the same as with other muscles of the body, the strength you require will depend largely on what activity and movement you would like to do. Of course, there is a level of strength that all women will require to maintain their pelvic health and not experience symptoms.

Understanding the key strength training principles will help you understand how to gain pelvic floor muscle strength. Sometimes when therapists prescribe pelvic floor muscle training programs (PFMT) there is little consideration to what it is we are aiming to achieve. Certainly, when you read about PFMT programs online, the general prescription is 10x10 second holds aiming for 3 sets. This however does not include the key components of strength training.

Strength training requires:

1. Maximal muscle contractions – meaning the strongest muscle contraction we can generate
2. For the muscles to reach fatigue
3. A repetition range of 8-12 maximum contractions at moderate velocity – holding for 10 seconds
4. 1-2 minutes rest between sets
5. An initial training frequency of 2-3 times per week, progressing to 3-4 days per week
6. Progressive muscle overload – with a 2 – 10% increase in load when the individual can perform 1-3 repetitions over the tar-

geted number (meaning when you can achieve 13 – 14 repetitions if aiming for 12, or 9-10 repetitions if aiming for 8 etc.)

If you are aiming to increase the strength of your pelvic floor muscles, and you can achieve 12 repetitions of maximal PFM contractions holding for 10 seconds, you will need to add some resistance.

There are several different types of strength training systems that you can use and I encourage you to do your research. My favourite system is the Aquaflex system available from http://pelvicfloorexercise.com.au/

The Aquaflex Pelvic Floor Exercise System consists of vaginal cones with adjustable weights to strengthen the pelvic floor muscles. The system can be used for strength and endurance training and can provide feedback as you use it during functional tasks. This system gives you an opportunity for a progressive program, provides great feedback because you can tell how long you can hold the weights and what weight you are using, plus they are functional - meaning you can use them in day-to-day activities.

Here are some examples of how the system can be used:

- Endurance training - holding the weighted cones in the vagina for periods to improve the endurance of the pelvic floor muscles.
- Resistance and strength training – using the weighted cones as additional resistance in pelvic floor strength training program/s.
- Feedback – using the weighted cones to provide feedback while doing functional activities like making the bed or emptying the dishwasher. You can progress to using them during

exercise to give feedback on when you should be contracting the pelvic floor muscles.

PELVIC FLOOR ENDURANCE

Muscular endurance is the ability of a muscle or group of muscles to sustain repeated contractions against resistance for an extended period of time. The resistance doesn't necessarily need to be a weight, and in the case of the pelvic floor can be our own body weight. Pelvic floor muscle endurance is required to get us to the end of the day feeling supported. Pelvic floor muscle endurance is also part of what is required to help us continue to feel supported and remain continent during a workout.

Endurance training differs from strength training, in that only light to moderate loads are required. Rather than doing maximal contractions, only 40-60% maximal contractions are needed. Higher repetitions (more than 15) and longer holds with a short rest of fewer than 90 seconds between sets is ideal. Endurance training programs are best done every other day.

Example of a pelvic floor endurance training program:

- Squeeze and lift the muscles of your pelvic floor to 50% of your maximal lift.
- To gauge a 'half-way lift' imagine your pelvic floor as an elevator moving from the ground level (completely relaxed) to level one (1), two (2), three (3) all the way to level five (5) which is a full lift.
- Once you are aware of how a full lift feels, imagine lifting to level three (3) only. This is a 'half-way lift'. For a full lift, relaxing only to halfway, imagine moving the elevator from level five (5) and relaxing only to level three (3).

- Hold the contraction for 30 seconds
- Relax for 15 seconds
- Repeat 15 times

PELVIC FLOOR CO-ORDINATION

As mentioned earlier, co-ordination of the pelvic floor muscles is required first to be able to contract fast enough to brace for a cough/sneeze (for example) and, secondly, to be able to sustain the contraction during the cough/sneeze. Co-ordination programs require a range of differently paced squeeze and rest periods. They require multiple sets per day, do not need to be maximal contractions, and do not require the muscles to reach a point of fatigue.

Here is an example of a co-ordination training program:

- Do 10 fast squeezes of the pelvic floor with no hold and rest-pause in between followed by;
- 10 slow squeezes with fast releases, followed by;
- 10 fast squeezes with a slow-release, followed by;
- Rest for one minute
- 5 half lifts (see previous description) with full relaxation
- 5 full lifts, relaxing only halfway in between

'THE KNACK'

The Knack is a term used to describe the 'bracing' of the pelvic floor before an activity that will increase intra-abdominal pressure such as a cough, a sneeze, or a laugh. Performing The Knack helps to support the pelvic organs including the bladder and the urethra in a position that allows them to overcome the intra-abdominal pressure created by the cough/sneeze/laugh. When performed at the right time and with enough strength, The Knack can stop or significantly reduce bladder leakage.

Essentially, 'The Knack' is a strong, well-timed contraction of the pelvic floor muscles. To use this technique contact the muscles of the pelvic floor strongly *before* and *during* times of increased intra-abdominal pressure (such as a cough/sneeze, laugh, heavy lift, or jump). For example, if you can sense you are about to sneeze, contract the muscles of the pelvic floor before you sneeze and continue to hold that contraction as you sneeze.

Repeating this technique often enough will create new neural pathways for some women, to the extent that they no longer need to think about it after some time. Other women will need to continue to consciously develop this habit as part of their lifestyle. Either way, when performed well, The Knack is known to significantly improve or stop bladder leakage entirely. It requires adequate strength, coordination, and sometimes endurance for multiple cough/s sneezes for it to be fully effective.

PELVIC FLOOR MUSCLE TRAINING TIPS

GET TO KNOW YOUR PELVIC FLOOR

The best way to develop a good understanding of the strength, coordination, and endurance of your pelvic floor muscles, as well as the condition of other pelvic support structures (such as ligaments and fascia), is to have an internal vaginal assessment with a pelvic floor physiotherapist. Some therapists will offer an ultrasound assessment rather than an internal vaginal exam but ultrasounds are much less accurate and offer far less information.

There are very few therapists who work with the pelvic floor on a physical *and* energetic/emotional level, but if you do find a therapist who does offer this type of holistic therapy and are interested in this approach, I highly recommend finding a therapist who has both a clinical physiological understanding of the pelvic floor, alongside the emotional and energetic core.

As well as seeing a pelvic floor physiotherapist, it's important to self-monitor your pelvic health. See the 'Pelvic Health Self Care' practices for more on this.

DO YOUR STRENGTH TRAINING AT NIGHT

If you are focusing on *strength training* it's recommended to do this at night or towards the end of the day. Remember, to gain strength it is required that you work your muscles to fatigue, you don't want to fatigue a pelvic floor that needs to support you all day. When strength training is done at night, or at least towards the end of the day, it gives your pelvic floor muscles an opportunity to rest overnight giving them a better chance to support you during the daytime when you are generally more active.

USE SIMPLE CUES

Evidence shows that the simplest cues to illicit pelvic floor muscle contractions are the best. According to the evidence, *the best cue* is "squeeze your anus". (Ben-Ami and Dar, 2018). This cue, however, leads us to focus on the deeper layer of the pelvic floor muscles only. In addition, you can use the cue squeeze around the vagina. Keeping the cue simple will give you a better chance of contracting the muscles effectively.

CONSIDER FEEDBACK TOOLS

There is a range of feedback tools on the market including the Aquaflex System and the Pelvic Floor Educator which is a device designed to help you know if you are contracting your pelvic floor muscles correctly. The Pelvic Floor Educator is designed to sit in the vagina and stay in place during use. As you contract your pelvic floor, the deep layer of pelvic floor muscles should shorten and lift. This movement lifts the probe in the vagina and the indicator stick moves downwards towards your tailbone - indicating a correct contraction. If you bear down instead (push down on the pelvic floor muscles, rather than lifting upwards and inwards) the stick will lift up and/or the probe will start to slide out if you are bearing down strongly. The external indicator stick amplifies this movement to show whether these muscles are being contracted correctly or not.

You can also use your own body to offer some feedback if you are doing your exercises effectively. These tools are not designed to be a replacement to a pelvic floor physiotherapy assessment, rather as an adjunct to treatment. Of course, you can choose not to seek pelvic floor physio and use these simple self-feedback tips instead, but they do not provide as much information as an internal vaginal assessment from a qualified therapist would.

SELF FEEDBACK TIPS

1. Insert a thumb or finger into the vagina, and then squeeze your pelvic floor muscles. You should feel the muscles drawing inward to squeeze around your thumb/finger, as well as a drawing upwards into the body.

2. Attempt to slow the flow of urine: as you urinate, attempt to stop the flow of urine. Generally, you won't stop it completely, but if you are activating the pelvic floor muscles correctly you should notice that the flow of urine slows.

3. Observe the perineum: the perineum is the body of tissue that sits between the vagina and the anus. Using a handheld mirror in a position where you can observe the perineum, squeeze the muscles of the pelvic floor. You should see the perineal body draw inward if you are activating your pelvic floor muscles correctly. If you notice

your perineum pushing outwards, you know that you are bearing down, rather than activating the muscles to draw inward and upward.

TROUBLESHOOTING PELVIC FLOOR MUSCLE (PFM) EXERCISES

If you are having difficulty sensing a PFM contraction, initiating a contraction, or finding it too challenging to maintain a contraction you can:

- Try a different position. Generally, the easier positions to activate the pelvic floor in are side-lying, four-point kneeling, or lying on your back. Sitting and standing can be more challenging.
- Check your alignment. Finding a relatively neutral position with the head stacked over the heart and the heart stacked over the pelvis with a neutral pelvic tilt may make it easier for you to initiate a pelvic floor contraction. Experiment with different positions and see how your body responds. (more on p. 173 - 175)
- Take a rest and try again later.
- Let the PFM relax with the breath in, and close and lift on the breath out - or vice versa. Trying something different is often useful.
- Seek help from a women's health physiotherapist.

YONI EGGS AND VAGINAL WEIGHTS

Yoni is the Sanskrit word for the female genitalia and reproductive organs. Yoni eggs are egg-shaped crystals that are specifically designed to place into the vagina for the purposes of healing, body connection, and strengthening the pelvic floor muscles. There is a range of crystals that are used to make Yoni eggs, the most common being jade, rose quartz, and black obsidian. Each of these crystals is said to have unique healing properties.

Jade: may help with bladder problems, menstrual difficulties, PMS, pregnancy, and childbirth. Note: *it is not* recommended to us any Yoni egg or feedback device during pregnancy due to the potential increased risk of bacterial vaginosis and increased risks during pregnancy.

Rose quartz: said to help with circulation, healing mothers after a complicated birth, fertility, the health of the female reproductive system, and healthy flow of fluids.

Black obsidian: is said to be useful to recover from trauma of any kind, in particular sexual assault. It is said to help express grief, and be useful in physical shock recovery.

(Eason, 2015).

There are a few key differences between Yoni eggs and other vaginal weights/feedback devices, the first being that feedback devices always (in my experience) have some type of string/cord that can be used to help remove the device whereas Yoni eggs only sometimes have one. In terms of safe use, and not needing to bear down to help to remove feedback tools including Yoni eggs, I would certainly recommend choosing an egg that is 'drilled' and does have a string/cord attached. Some Yoni eggs are advertised as being able to be worn during intercourse, which I would strongly caution against. Another key difference is the healing properties of Yoni egg crystals. Depending on your beliefs, you may prefer to choose an egg as opposed to other devices because of the innate healing properties of each crystal. In my opinion one is not necessarily superior to another, it is just dependent on what you feel is right for you.

PELVIC FLOOR RELAXATION

Breathing deep into the Pelvic Bowl, as you do in the Deep Core Connection Practice is a beautiful way to bring relaxation into the pelvic floor. Pelvic floor self-massage is another practice within this book dedicated to pelvic floor relaxation.

If you do experience pelvic pain, or if you suspect you have pelvic tension or an overactive pelvic floor, bring a simple awareness to your pelvic floor during the day to check in with your pelvic floor and invite your muscles to soften and relax. You may wish to set repeating reminders on your phone to help you remember. It can be surprising how much and how often we can be over-activating the muscles of the pelvic floor and generating unnecessary tension within the deep core. Good times to check-in and monitor deep core and pelvic floor tension are during simple tasks like brushing your teeth and washing the dishes.

The following stretches may also be beneficial if you experience pelvic tension or suspect you have 'overactive' pelvic floor muscles. Please keep in mind that some of these poses/stretches may require modification during pregnancy. The following poses may cause a stretching sensation, but should never cause pain. Gentle stretching is more beneficial than forceful stretching, as the body will remain calm and relaxed with a more gentle approach. Pushing into pain will only cause the muscles to resist the stretch, causing the opposite of the desired effect.

INNER THIGH STRETCHES

Women who experience pelvic floor tension often have tight muscles surrounding the hip joint. Stretching the muscles of the inner thighs, the glutes and the hip flexors can help.

FROGGY STRETCH

The pelvic floor and inner thighs are closely related. Stretching into the hips and the glutes can offer much relief and create a sense of spaciousness within the pelvic bowl.

This stretch can be very intense, and I recommended that you use supports to allow you to relax into this position without creating a strain on the muscles. It's important when we stretch that we allow ourselves to fully relax, otherwise, we will be adding to muscle tension rather than helping to release, relieve, and relax the muscles.

- Begin by sitting on the feet with the knees wide.
- Reach your arms forward using them to support you as you bring your chest to rest on your support – a bolster or a rolled blanket.
- Gently bring the feet and knees a little wider.
- Once you feel a gentle stretch simply relax and rest in this position.
- You can play with stretching different parts of your muscle by shifting your pelvis further from or closer towards your feet. A gentle rocking motion may feel nice.
- You can also stretch different muscle fibres by rocking the pelvis into a more anterior (forward tilting) or posterior (backward) pelvic tilt – as opposed to moving further from or closer to the feet, you are simply changing the *tilt* of the pelvis.
- Come out of this position in the opposite way that you came into it.

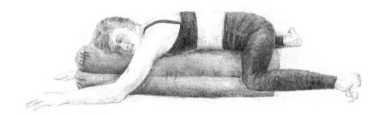

DEEP SQUAT

- Take the legs wider than the hips and turn the toes out.
- Bring yourself into a deep squat pose. If you find this challenging, raise the heels a little bit by placing them on a rolled-up towel.
- Take your hands to meet at the front of your chest and either interlace the fingers to clasp the hands together or create a prayer position with the hands
- Use the elbows or side of your arms to press against the knees/inner thighs to create an additional stretch.

From this position, you can take the hands to the floor to support you and stretch one leg out long to the side to change to a DEEP SIDE LUNGE. To intensify the stretch, continue to use your arm to provide a gentle overpressure to the bent leg pushing backward.

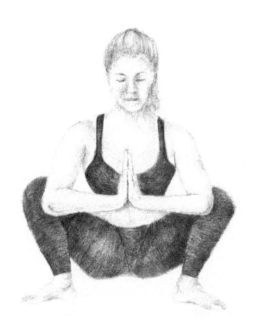

HAPPY BABY POSE

- Lay on your back.
- Bring your legs into a tabletop position.

- Take your knees wider than your armpits and gently hug the knees towards your chest so that you can grasp your inner foot, your ankles, or take the index and middle fingers to wrap around your big toes.
- Use your hands to gently pull the feet downwards to create a stretch at the inner thighs.
- Press your sacrum onto the ground.
- You can hold this as a static pose or gently rock from side to side in this position.

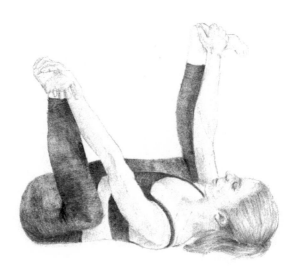

BUTTERFLY POSE

- In a sitting position, let the knees fall open and let the soles of the feet touch.
- For additional stretch clasp the ankles with your hands and use the elbows and forearms to press the knees towards the floor.
- Take a gentle lean forward to increase the intensity of the pose.

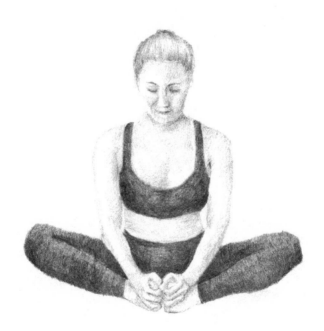

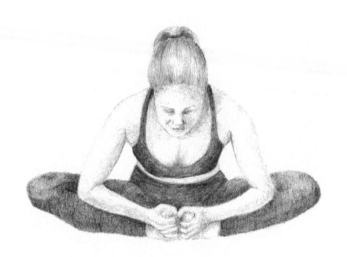

GLUTE STRETCHES

GLUTE FIGURE 4 STRETCH

- Start by lying on your back with the knees bent and feet resting on the floor.
- Lift one leg to bring one foot to rest on the opposite knee.
- Lift the other foot into a tabletop position.
- You should feel a stretch of the glutes.
- To increase the stretch, you can thread one hand between your legs and the other to wrap around the outside of your leg

to grasp just below the knee or shin. Use your arms to hug the legs in towards your body.

- Alter the amount of bend in the leg that you are stretching and the position of your foot on your thigh to stretch different muscle fibres.

This stretch can also be performed sitting or standing.

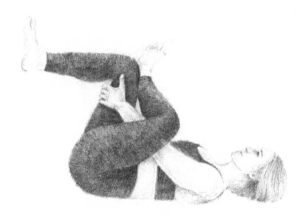

GLUTES SEPARATION

Women who experience pelvic floor tension often do this intuitively. It is as simple as using both hands to grasp between the buttocks and pull the flesh of the glutes away from one another to create space between the buttocks. Preferred positions to do this in are usually standing or laying in your back with the legs about hip-distance apart, the knees bent, and feet flat on the floor.

QUAD STRETCHES

QUAD KNEELING POSE

- Take a kneeling position with your left foot forward.
- Support your body with both hands on your left knee.
- Step your left foot slightly further away from your supporting knee.
- Lean forward to deepen your lunge, keeping your hips square and tilting your pubic bone upwards.
- To deepen the stretch, you can take your right hand and twist back to reach for your right foot. Gently draw your right foot towards your buttocks. Continue to keep the hips square and tuck your tailbone under so that you feel a stretch in the front of your hips.

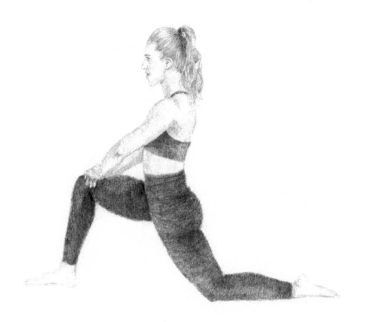

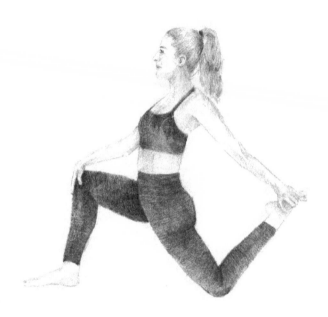

QUAD STRETCH IN SIDE LYING POSITION:

- Laying on your side with your legs long, keep a gentle bend in your knees to support you.
- Stack your hips and legs on top of one another.
- Bend your top knee and take a hold of your foot or ankle.
- Gently pull your foot towards your buttocks.
- Continue to maintain the alignment of your pelvis, pressing your pubic bone forward so that you feel a stretch in the front of your hip.

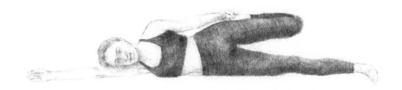

SUPPORTED BRIDGE

- Lie on your back with your knees bent and your feet flat.
- Walk your feet back towards your buttocks.
- If you have a block, press your hips towards the roof and bring the block under the sacrum to support you. You can choose what side of the block you use, depending on your flexibility and how deep you want to stretch.
- Hold this position, aiming to feel a gentle stretch at the front of the thighs.

- Alternatively, bring the low or medium edge of your block, a bolster, or a couple of rolled towels/blankets to rest under the sacrum, and then stretch the legs and arms long to feel at stretch at the front of the hips.

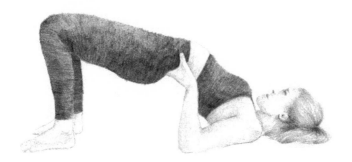

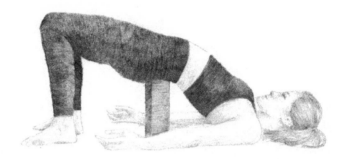

LEGS UP THE WALL POSE:

This is a beautiful pose to help to relax and restore the pelvic floor. You may enjoy the sensation of increased blood flow in the pelvic bowl in this position. Women with pelvic organ prolapse symptoms or high tone pelvic floor muscles may find this a relieving position. This is also a nice position to practice pelvic bowl breathing.

- Start by sitting quite closely and side onto a wall, then move into a position such that you are laying on your side with the legs slightly bent and remaining alongside the wall.

- Roll yourself gently onto your back, and let the legs rest long against the wall. You may wish to use a support such as a block/bolster/pillow/folded towel or blanket to support under the lower back or hips.
- Rest in this position for about 5-10 minutes or as long as it feels good for you.
- Take your time as you move out of this position, particularly when coming back to standing as the change in blood pressure may cause light-headedness or dizziness.

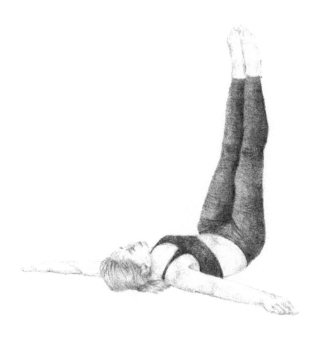

RESTORING THE DEEP CORE
THROUGH MOVEMENT

What impacts your core function during movement?

There is a whole range of things that will impact how the core functions during a particular task, movement, or activity including:
The task itself:

- The position/posture required for the task
- Duration of load/weight/impact – this relates to the 'fatigability' of the muscles.
- The level of impact/weight/load during the task
- The speed of a task and the ability of the muscles to contract/relax and respond accordingly

Your unique musculoskeletal system:

- Your unique posture/position that you adopt to perform the task
- The ability of the core muscles to contract and relax
- The flexibility, strength, coordination, and endurance of the deep core muscles as well as other muscles required to perform the task
- The condition of the body's soft tissues including the ligaments and fascia that support the pelvic organs
- How you breathe during that task
- Your core strategy - how you use your core as a whole

This is why an individualised approach to exercise is required with consideration of the integrity and overall function of the deep core and pelvic floor, your preferred movement patterns, as well as your unique values, vision, and goals.

There are some common tendencies that we have when approaching exercise that can cause 'core imbalances'. These tendencies generally relate to either: over-activating the muscles, not engaging the muscles strong enough, or not contracting the muscles early enough or for long enough during a particular movement. The ABCDE approach is designed to help you to understand how to engage your core effectively during movement, as well as how to monitor, modify and progress your movement accordingly.

In the ABCDE approach:
A = Alignment
B = Breath
C = Core
D = Do it
E = Evaluate
The purpose of the ABCDE approach towards movement is to help you:

- Find ways to move your body that help to rebuild deep core strength, endurance and coordination
- Bring awareness to your deep core and pelvic floor during movement
- Explore movement and reduce the risk of developing deep core or pelvic floor symptoms during movement
- Improve symptoms of pelvic organ prolapse or stress urinary incontinence caused by particular types of movement
- Find an appropriate starting point for your movement from which you can progress

- Increase confidence in your body's strength and natural support systems

When using the ABCDE approach to movement, it's important to understand that we all have different ways in which we prefer moving our body, and that there is no one right way to move your body. This approach to movement is designed to help you explore your own body and experiment with movement using evidence-based principles that can help you to engage your deep core effectively.

ALIGNMENT

Muscles can generate the most force when they are in a relatively neutral alignment. Therefore, positioning our body with relatively neutral alignment helps the muscles of the deep core to contract most strongly during movement. It may be helpful to imagine the core as a canister. To maintain a neutral posture, avoid 'kinking' the canister during your movement.

To achieve a neutral posture, first experiment in standing:

- Notice your feet, and where you feel the weight in your feet. Is your weight at the front of your foot, at your heels, or does your weight feel like it is evenly spread over the entire foot? If you feel your weight is more in the front or rear of your foot, gently transition your weight so that you feel the weight distributed more evenly in the foot.
- Next, bring your attention to your pelvic position. Gently tilt the pelvis forwards and backward until you find somewhere in the middle. The midline position is not an exact spot but simply a position where you don't feel that the pelvis is tilted

forward or tucked under. To help you to tilt your pelvis, you may need to bend your knees slightly.

- Then bring your awareness to your rib cage, and feel that your rib cage is stacked over your pelvis.
- Then bring your awareness to the rib cage itself, and find a midline position of the ribcage. To do this, bring your awareness to your breath, and sense where your breath is directed when you inhale deeply. In a neutral posture, your breath will flow into the rib cage and the belly quite evenly. If you feel your breath is directed solely into the rib cage, your rib cage is likely flared open. In this case gently draw your rib cage to close a little, bringing your nipples downward a little, and your breast bone more towards your pubic bone. If you feel that your breath flows into the belly only, it is likely that you are in a more hunched over position. To bring yourself into a more neutral posture, gently lift the rib cage to open, lifting the nipples upward a little, and lifting the breastbone away from the pubic bone. Place one hand on the outside of the rib cage and one hand on the belly to feel how the breath changes as you change your posture.
- When you have done each of these steps, scan back over your body to feel if you have lost any of your postural changes.

Using the above practice helps you to find a neutral position in standing. In a static standing posture it is helpful to feel the weight evenly in your feet to find a neutral posture. In terms of movement, however, your weight distribution on your feet will change depending on what movement you are performing, and will become less important to focus on. It is the position of your rib cage stacked over your pelvis, along with the neutral position of the rib cage and pelvis itself that you will find more useful.

Remember, using a neutral posture is designed to help with the activation of the muscles of the deep core. As you become stronger and more confident in your movement, it's ideal to experiment with movement in many different postures and patterns. For certain types of movement, like heavy lifting for example, you may want to maintain your neutral posture always while when performing other forms of movement, it will be less important. The key is to become aware of your own body, and experiment with how different movement patterns feel for you and how they impact your deep core and any pelvic floor symptoms you may experience. Some women find that by changing their posture alone, they can significantly reduce symptoms of prolapse or incontinence during exercise.

BREATH

Your breath is one of the most powerful ways that you can control the pressure within the deep core. When you are breathing in a relaxed state you may notice the breath expanding the rib cage, the belly bulging, and the pelvic floor softening.

You can use your breath to help you determine if you are achieving and maintaining a neutral posture by assessing where your breath tends to flow during your movement. In a neutral posture, the breath will flow quite evenly to expand the lower ribs and bulge the belly. If your rib cage is open or flared, you will notice the breath flow more so into the rib cage, and not into the belly. The upper chest will tend to move more as it fills with air as well. If you have a more hunched thoracic position, you will likely see the breath flow more so into the belly. Shifting the position of your rib cage to achieve a more neutral alignment (as described in the alignment practice above) will help you to find an even flow of breath. In this way, you are using your breath as a form of feedback to help you find a neutral posture.

You can also use your breath to help mitigate the pressure within the deep core. Breathing out on exertion is one way you can do this. With certain exercises you may find that you need to exhale in more than one part of the exercise. Take a squat, for example. You may sense you need to breathe out on the knee bend, as well as on the return back to standing. What you perceive to be the harder component of a particular exercise may be specific to you. Therefore, breathing out on the component of the exercise that you feel is most challenging makes more sense than breathing in/out on someone else's cue. During impact exercises, like box jumps for example, you may find it helpful to exhale on the landing.

You can also use your breath to help guide how challenging an exercise is for you. Exercises that require us to brace and hold our breath tend to be exercises that significantly increase our intra-abdominal pressure. While breath-holding isn't an incorrect strategy, you may choose not to perform exercises that require breath holds during times when we want to be protective of our deep core, like in the early postpartum period or at times when you anticipate prolapse symptoms to become worse.

CORE

As mentioned earlier, core imbalances tend to occur when we either over-activate the muscles of the deep core during movement or don't engage the core strongly enough, swiftly enough, or for long enough. It can be challenging to know if you are contracting your deep core and pelvic floor too strongly, or not effectively enough, because they lead to similar symptoms such as incontinence. Bearing down, or pushing onto the pelvic floor rather than squeezing and lifting is another challenge that some women have when attempting to engage the deep core. This happens in about 15-20% of women. The best way to be sure you are activating the muscles of the pelvic floor correctly is to seek an assessment from a women's health/pelvic floor physiotherapist. If you are unable to see a pelvic floor physio-therapist, or choose not to, you can use the guidance offered in the self-feedback of the pelvic floor on page 153. The following guid-ance can be used either alongside your self-assessment, or the guid-ance from your therapist. Experimenting with core contraction (by increasing the strength of the contraction, or allowing the muscles to soften) can give you more information about what is required to reduce symptoms during movement.

Just like any other muscle group, the amount of force that needs to be generated by the deep core will depend on the task itself. If you were to pick up a pen from a desk, the amount of force you gener-ate through your arm would be much less than if you were lifting a child. This same principle pertains to the muscles of the deep core. The degree of deep core contraction will depend on the task. There are a couple of reasons why you want to avoid over-contracting the muscles of the deep core during movement.

- It causes the muscles to fatigue prematurely, making them less capable of maintaining support for the entirety of an exercise program.
- Gripping the muscles of the abdomen, which many women tend to do, doesn't allow intra-abdominal pressure to be evenly spread across the deep core. This can put unnecessary force downward onto the pelvic floor and contribute to in-continence and prolapse symptoms.
- Over-activation of muscles may cause muscular imbalances that may lead to pain.

To avoid over-activating the muscles of the deep core:

- Simply think about matching your deep core tension to the movement that you are performing.
- Allow yourself to breathe into your belly.
- Use the 'spread the load' concept explained below.

'Spreading the load' is a concept to visualise during movement or exercise that helps to encourage activation of the deep core without overdoing it. As you contract the deep core and pelvic floor in preparation for a task, you then imagine 'spreading the load' throughout your body. 'The load' refers to any part of your body where you feel the intensity. For example, this could mean imagining the energy of the contraction you feel at the deep core and spreading it across the entire body, or it might refer to sensing the load of a bar before a lift, and spreading the load across the chest, through the body and into the legs. There is no one right way to use this concept. Instead, it is a visualisation that can be applied to any movement.

In some instances, the deep core won't activate strongly enough to provide and maintain adequate support for a particular task. This can lead to musculoskeletal injury, pelvic floor symptoms, and in the presence of DRAM (separation of the abdominal muscles) 'doming' of the abdomen and a lack of tension at the Linea Alba (the connective tissue between the rectus abdominal muscles). In this case, activating the deep core before the desired movement and being mindful to maintain the contraction throughout the task may be helpful.

DO IT

Do it means exactly that - perform the task. In my opinion, when you are experimenting with a type of movement that you would like to perform, it's best to start with the easiest form of that movement and progress until you find a point in which you feel that you are being challenged by the movement but not pushing your body beyond it's 'safe zone'. 'Do it' is about experimenting with your body, finding your edge, challenging yourself, being honest with yourself, and meeting yourself where you are.

As you perform the movement task, evaluate how your body responds.

EVALUATE

As you perform a task or movement, maintain awareness in the body. Be aware of any pelvic symptoms that you notice during the movement, and monitor for doming of the abdomen if you have concerns with abdominal separation. Be aware that sometimes pelvic symptoms such as heaviness, dragging, or pelvic pain may not be present during a particular exercise but may develop in the hours afterward. Just because you don't notice symptoms during or straight away after the movement, it doesn't mean the movement wasn't the cause or perhaps a contributing factor of the symptoms. If you have pelvic symptoms, or if you are experimenting with new kinds of movement, I recommend doing a small amount and then monitoring your how your body responds both during the movement itself and in the 24-48 hours afterward. If no symptoms develop, then you may choose to progress your movement/exercise while remembering that no symptoms doesn't necessarily mean there is no change to the pelvic floor. If you do develop symptoms during a movement, stop and modify the movement to make it easier. If you have a delayed onset of symptoms, or symptoms that linger, wait until they resolve before experimenting again with the movement that aggravated the symptoms. Once the symptoms have resolved you may choose to continue to experiment with a modification of the movement that you know or suspect caused the concerns.

As you evaluate how your body responds to movement, you then maintain the current movement or modify the movement accordingly. There are many ways that you can change how you are moving your body to make the movement easier or more challenging. The idea of using the ABCDE technique is that you can 'troubleshoot' your movement by being aware of your alignment, your breath, and your core strategy to find how you might change your movement pattern to help to prevent and/or resolve any symptoms you may be experiencing or at risk of. In addition, there are many other things that you can modify to make movement harder or easier including:

- Changing the speed of your movement. It's a common misconception that slowing down movement *always* makes a task easier. This is not the case. Sometimes slowing down your movement can make it more challenging. Generally though, slowing down your pace is a good way to modify your movement if you are experiencing challenges with your deep core or pelvic floor.
- Modifying the load. Think broadly when it comes to reducing the load of an exercise. Reducing the load doesn't always refer to reducing the amount of external weight you are resisting during a movement. It may also refer to reducing the amount of gravitational pull created by movement. Changing your position can reduce the gravitational pull on the body - for example, squats on a Pilates reformer can offer a reduced load compared to squats in a standing position because gravity is acting differently on the body. Another way to reduce load is to immerse yourself in water. Water depth impacts the load placed on the body in differing degrees depending on the depth of immersion. Of course, to make an exercise or movement pattern more challenging, weight can be added.

- Modifying the duration, either by reducing the number of repetitions/time spent performing a particular task, and/or increasing the rest time between sets or repetitions,
- Modifying the range of the movement. To make a movement easier, reduce the range of movement. Alternatively, to make the movement more advanced, increase the range. Increasing the depth of a squat, or bringing your legs wider apart, for example, will increase the difficulty while decreasing the depth of the squat, and keeping the legs closer together will make the squat easier.

5

PREGNANCY, BIRTH, AND
BEYOND

In this first section of Pregnancy, Birth, and Beyond, I will talk more to the physical aspects of pregnancy, birth, and postpartum recovery. In the later part of this section, I will offer thoughts around pregnancy, birth, and motherhood from a more emotional and energetic perspective.

When it comes to the deep core through pregnancy, birth, and beyond much of our focus tends to be on the physical changes that occur and what we need to do to optimise our deep core health during these transition phases. There are significant physical deep core and pelvic floor changes during these times, and we don't often give attention and respect to the degree of change that our bodies go through during pregnancy and birth. Without giving ourselves time to understand and get to know our body during these transitions, we can feel like strangers in our own homes. Reigniting your connection with your physical, emotional, energetic, and spiritual body beyond birth creates and nurtures the essential foundational components of our relationship with self.

EXERCISE DURING PREGNANCY

During pregnancy, we tend to be quite good at looking after our physical health because we are focused on creating an optimal environment for our baby to grow and thrive. Sometimes though, in trying to create a particular environment, we create new levels of anxiety for ourselves.

Being a pelvic floor therapist, one of the huge concerns that I hear about from women is knowing how to safely exercise during pregnancy and I see a range of mindsets in approaching exercise during pregnancy. Some women become scared and perhaps overly cautious and concerned about exercise, whereas others who feel very confident and comfortable exercising can have little consideration of the effects of exercise on their deep core and pelvic floor during pregnancy.

Historically, in the early to mid-1900s it was believed that exercise during pregnancy was not safe and that it should be discouraged. Over time as new evidence emerged, it became known that exercise during pregnancy is usually safe and should be encouraged. There is overwhelmingly good evidence to support exercise during pregnancy. The American College of Obstetricians and Gynaecologists have collated evidence-based guidelines for exercise during pregnancy stating that:

- Physical activity and exercise in pregnancy are associated with minimal risks and have been shown to benefit most women, although some modification to exercise routines may be necessary because of normal anatomical and physiological changes and foetal requirements.
- Women with uncomplicated pregnancies should be encouraged to engage in aerobic and strength-conditioning exercises before, during, and after pregnancy.
- A thorough clinical evaluation should be conducted before recommending an exercise program to ensure that a patient does not have a medical reason to avoid exercise.
- Obstetrician-gynaecologists and other obstetric care providers should carefully evaluate women with medical or obstetric complications before making recommendations on physical activity participation during pregnancy. Activity restriction should not be prescribed routinely as a treatment to reduce preterm birth.
- Additional research is required to study the effects of exercise on pregnancy-specific conditions and outcomes and to clarify further effective behavioural counselling methods and the op-

timal type, frequency, and intensity of exercise. Similar research is needed to create an improved evidence base concerning the effects of occupational physical activity on maternal-foetal health.

- An exercise program that leads to an eventual goal of moderate-intensity exercise for at least 20-30 minutes (150 minutes per week) on most if not all days in the week should be developed. The use of ratings of perceived exertion (RPE) is perhaps the most effective means of monitoring moderate exercise intensity during pregnancy compared to heart rate parameters. For moderate-intensity exercise, the RPE should be 13-14 on the Modified Borg Scale. [An image of the Modified Borg Scale is readily available on the internet, via a Google search. Using the "talk test" is another way to measure your rate of perceived exertion. As long as you can maintain a conversation while you exercise, you are not likely to be overexerting yourself.]

- Regular physical activity during pregnancy increases the probability of vaginal delivery, maintains physical fitness, and helps with weight management. It reduces the risk of gestational diabetes, gestational hypertensive disorders (defined as gestational hypertension or preeclampsia) preterm birth, caesarean section, and lower birth weight.

(The American College of Obstetricians and Gynecologists, 2020).

Of course, there are certain instances where exercise during pregnancy is absolutely contraindicated. There are also circumstances where exercise needs to be carefully monitored and professionally prescribed with an individualised approach.

Absolute contraindications to exercise during pregnancy include the following conditions:

- Haemodynamically significant heart disease
- Restrictive lung disease
- Severe anaemia
- Premature labour during the current pregnancy
- Ruptured membranes
- Multiple gestations at risk for premature delivery
- Persistent 2nd or 3rd trimester bleeding
- Incompetent cervix/cerclage
- Placenta Previa after 26 weeks gestation
- Pregnancy-induced hypertension / Preeclampsia

High-risk pregnancies where exercise should be individually prescribed and carefully monitored include short cervix and gestational diabetes.

According to the ACOG Guidelines (2020) the following activities are considered to be safe to initiate or continue during pregnancy:

- Walking
- Dancing
- Stationary cycling
- Aerobic exercises
- Resistance exercises (e.g. using weights, elastic bands)
- Stretching exercises
- Hydrotherapy, water aerobics

Things to be aware of about the above activities are:

- Yoga positions that result in a decreased venous return and hypotension (low blood pressure) should be avoided as much as possible.
- Motionless postures, such as certain yoga positions laying on your back (for example, Legs Up The Wall Pose), may result in decreased venous return and hypotension in 10-20% of all pregnant women and it is therefore recommended they are avoided as much as possible.
- In consultation with an obstetric care provider, running or jogging, racquet sports, and strength training may be safe for pregnant women who participated in these activities regularly before pregnancy.
- Racquet sports wherein a pregnant woman's changing balance may affect rapid movements and increase the risk of falling should be avoided as much as possible.
- 32 degrees Celsius is the maximum recommended temperature for water exercise while pregnant.
- Sweating is greater in swimming than running, so it is important to maintain hydration during water exercise.

In terms of overall body function, the following act as warning signs to cease exercise during pregnancy:

- Vaginal bleeding
- Regular painful contractions/preterm labour
- Shortness of breath before commencing exercise
- Dizziness
- Headache
- Chest pain

- Calf pain or calf swelling
- Amniotic fluid leakage
- Muscle weakness affecting balance

In terms of the deep core and pelvic floor function, the following act as warning signs to cease exercise during pregnancy and modify accordingly:

- Incontinence
- Low back pain
- Pelvic or vaginal heaviness
- Any sensation of direct downward pressure onto the pelvic floor
- Doming or 'tenting' of the abdomen *may* lead to increased separation of the abdominal muscles

DEEP CORE AND PELVIC FLOOR CHANGES DURING PREGNANCY

While all women experience different pregnancies, there are common changes that happen to a woman's body when she is pregnant.

POSTURAL CHANGES DURING PREGNANCY

Due to how we carry our babies there are some common changes that we notice in our posture including:

- Shifting the rib cage behind the pelvis
- Increase/change in position of the natural curves in the spine
- Rib cage 'flares' and widens

Some women will notice their pelvic position changes too. Commonly, a posterior pelvic tilt or a 'bum tuck' will occur during pregnancy. Sometimes these postural changes continue postpartum, which may contribute to ongoing musculoskeletal and pelvic health concerns. These changes may not cause specific concerns or pain, but may simply cause us to feel different in our body after birth. This is just one reason why it's important to take time to reconnect and get to know your body after birth.

ABDOMINAL SEPARATION

There are several names given to the separation of the abdominal muscles including diastasis, rectus diastasis, and diastasis rectus abdominal muscle or 'DRAM'. Over the past few years, education and awareness of diastasis have increased. While increasing awareness is welcomed, the hype that comes with it is not always helpful. Some women are led to believe that they have something wrong with their body, when in fact this separation is a normal occurrence and happens in 100% of pregnancies. (Lee, 2017)

The separation occurs at the Linea Alba, which is the name given to the connective tissue that holds the rectus muscles together. During pregnancy, as baby grows, the connective tissue is stretched causing the separation to occur. Shortly after birth, some women will have a smaller separation of just 1-2 fingers in width, while other women will have wider separations. There are reports that some women are genetically predisposed to a wider separation. Though we have many theories as to the contributing factors of a larger separation for some women we have limited concrete evidence. There is generally a collective agreement amongst therapists that certain exercises should be avoided during pregnancy to help reduce the risk of contributing to a wider diastasis, but much of our education on this topic is based on anecdotal evidence or clinical hypothesis.

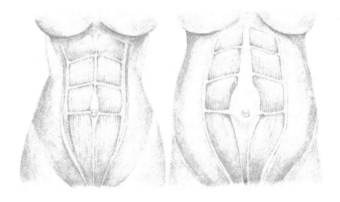

DIASTASIS

In terms of reducing the risk of increased abdominal separation, it is suggested that exercises that cause 'tenting' or 'doming' of the abdomen should be avoided during pregnancy. Exercises that signif- icantly increase intraabdominal pressure and increase the load of the abdominal muscles specifically are also generally not advised. Such exercises include:

- Sit-ups
- Plank positions
- Double leg lift/lowers
- Chin-ups
- Strong abdominal poses such as Boat Pose in yoga

While smaller separations will tend to heal without any specific exercise/therapy, larger separations may require specific exercise and intervention. Reasons for intervention may be cosmetic, in the sense that women simply do not like the appearance of their abdomen. For other women, it may be that the separation causes or contributes to other musculoskeletal concerns such as low back and pelvic pain, hernias, or other pelvic health concerns relating to bladder or bowel health or sexual function.

ASSESSMENT OF DRAM

Determining the presence of DRAM is not particularly difficult, yet many practitioners do not assess the entire length of the Linea Alba, or ignore the importance of being able to create tension across the Linea Alba. Ideally, an appropriately trained health professional can provide you with the following information:

- The presence or absence of a separation
- The length and width of the separation
- The depth of the separation
- If tension can be created across the Linea Alba

If you have not had access to an appropriate or accurate assessment, you can ask a partner or friend to assess for you. Though the assessment is simple, there is a skill in knowing what structures are being palpated, and what they feel like in the presence or absence of abdominal separation.

To assess for DRAM:

- Lay flat on your back with no pillow under the head
- The knees can be comfortably bent with the hips and feet supported, or legs stretched out long
- Ensure the entire length of the Linea Alba is exposed so that it can be seen and felt – from the sternum to the pubic bone
- Tuck your chin to your chest, and gently curl up
- The assessor uses their fingers to feel along the entire length of the Linea Alba feeling for any area where the muscles feel separated from one another, as well as feeling for the level of tension that is created along the Linea Alba. It is important to feel across the entire length of the Linea Alba as the separation can occur anywhere along its length.
- When feeling for tension, the assessor is feeling if the midline of the abdomen can create a firm tension that would feel similar to the firmness of cartilage at the tip on the nose, or if inadequate tension can be produced, which would feel more like pressing into a soft cheek.
- As you curl up, the assessor may feel the muscles 'coming together'.
- Feeling for the length, depth, and width of the separation in this curled position, along with how soft or firm the tissue feels, gives you the information you are seeking.

When the length and depth of any existing separation are established, and the in/ability to create tension is known, the second part of the assessment can take place.

Part Two of the assessment is to cue either a pelvic floor lift (squeeze the anus) or a transverse abdominis contraction (draw the belly button towards the spine) and then conduct the chin tuck. The assessor now feels for the tension at the Linea Alba to see if adequate tension (a firm feeling) can be created. If not, more practice may be required or more information such as pelvic floor function would be needed. In this case, while the exercises in this book may be helpful, I would suggest seeking personalised advice from a pelvic floor physiotherapist.

If you can 'close the gap' and create adequate tension across the Linea Alba, this exercise then becomes part of your training. Using whatever cue you find helpful, practice doing small curl-ups to create and maintain the tension at the midline of the abdomen.

TREATMENT OF DRAM

The treatment of DRAM is multifaceted and sometimes more complex than others. A personalised and individual approach to therapy is ideal particularly in more complex scenarios, but a generalised program with the exercises suggested here and further in this section may be helpful.

In terms of DRAM, there are a few key areas of focus for treatment:

1. Bringing the muscles 'together'
2. Improving the recruitment of the deep abdominal muscles so that they can create tension across the Linea Alba

3. Restoring the balance and co-ordination the muscles of the deep core

A combined treatment plan that encapsulates each of these key treatment focus points is recommended. The exercise mentioned above will be helpful, particularly if tension can be created across the midline of the abdomen. There are also postural positions that are thought to contribute to ongoing pressure at the midline of the abdomen, and therefore may potentially contribute to ongoing muscle separation.

If you take a look at the slumped posture on page 197, you can see that the woman's rib cage is positioned behind her pelvis, and her pelvis is in a posterior pelvic tilt position. Imagine the pressure on the abdomen for this woman. Compared to a neutral posture you can sense how the slumped posture depicted (p. 197) may contribute to continued diastasis. The first posture shows a classic 'military posture' where the woman's rib cage is flared wide and her pelvis in an anterior pelvic tilt position. This position can also potentially contribute to continued diastasis due to the increased stretch placed on the abdomen over time. I share this with caution because no posture is wrong. However, if we spend long periods in one particular position, it can create pressure on different parts of our body, as well as cause some muscles to become more active than others, and some to become less active.

A neutral posture helps to create a position that provides an opportunity for muscles to be working in a more balanced way and can reduce the pressure on the diastasis. By no means does this mean that you need to have perfect posture all the time but creating an awareness of your posture and position can help you to realise how much time you may spend in a particular position, and invite you to create more opportunities to spend time in different postures, either through movement practices, or simple body awareness practices.

To find a neutral posture start in a standing position.

- Notice your feet, and where you feel the weight in your feet. Is your weight at the front of your foot, at your heels, or does your weight feel like it is evenly spread over the entire foot? If you feel your weight is more in the front or rear of your foot, gently transition your weight so that you feel the weight distributed more evenly in the foot.
- Next, bring your attention to your pelvic position. Gently tilt the pelvis forwards and backward until you find somewhere in the middle. The midline position is not an exact spot, but simply a position where you don't feel that the pelvis is tilted forward or tucked under.
- Then, bring your awareness to your rib cage, and feel that your rib cage is stacked over your pelvis. Then bring your awareness to the rib cage itself, and find a midline position of the rib cage. To do this, bring your awareness to your breath, and sense where your breath is directed when you inhale deeply. In a neutral posture, your breath will flow into the rib cage and the belly. If you feel your breath is directed solely into the rib cage, your rib cage is likely flared open. In this case gently draw your rib cage to close a bit, bringing your nipples downward a little, and your breast bone more towards your pubic bone. If you feel that your breath flows into the belly only, it is likely that you are in a more hunched over position. To bring yourself into a more neutral posture, gently lift the rib cage to open, lifting the nipples upward a little, and lifting the breastbone away from the pubic bone. Place one hand on

the outside of the rib cage and one hand on the belly to feel how the breath changes as you change your posture.

- When you have done each of these steps, scan back over your body to feel if you have lost any of the postural adjustments you have made.

Once you have found your neutral position, sense how that feels in your body. For some, it will feel quite natural, for others it will feel like they are positioned in an extreme forward lean even though they are standing upright, and others feel like they have to work hard in their glutes to maintain a neutral pelvic position. Noticing what feels different to you will help you to know how you may like to challenge your posture throughout your day so that you can practice bringing your body into a position that counteracts your preferred posture.

Challenging and changing your posture takes focused effort over time. Bringing your awareness to your posture at multiple points during the day, and challenging yourself to adopt a position that feels different in your body is more helpful than trying to 'fix' your posture to be a certain way all the time. Posture is not meant to be static, nor is there one right way to hold yourself.

Strengthening muscles that tend to be less active is also helpful to bring balance into the body and gift yourself more opportunity to relax the pressure on muscles that tend to be dominant.

Practicing movement where tension is maintained across the Linea Alba is also helpful. To give a complete program of exercises and their progressions go beyond the scope of this book but with an understanding of your body, an openness to experiment with movement, and by using the ABCDE technique described on pages 172 - 181, it's possible to establish appropriate exercise modifications and progressions for yourself.

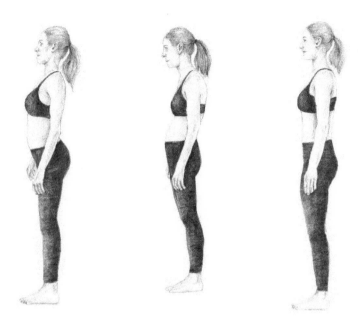

Abdominal support garments or abdominal compression garments are sometimes prescribed to help support the recovery of DRAM. When considering support/compression garments it is important to consider their possible effect on the pelvic floor. Postpartum garments are designed to give additional support to the abdomen, helping to decrease the load on the Linea Alba. In this way, support garments may aid the recovery of DRAM. However, additional pressure onto the deep core may increase the pressure onto the pelvic floor. Remembering the core is a canister and acts as a pressure system. The additional abdominal compression, along with gravity and the shape of the pelvic bowl, you may be able to visualise how a compression garment around the abdomen may create an additional downward pressure onto the pelvic floor – just like squeezing an upside down tube of toothpaste. Compression garments are not wrong, and in many instances may be helpful. Depending on what the 'weakest link' is within the deep core, abdominal binders may be helpful or could be potentially harmful. If a diastasis is the main concern, an abdominal binder may be a good option. However, if abdominal separation is combined with a pelvic floor concern, I would suggest avoiding the use of compression garments. It is important to consider, though, what your main concern is. The best way to know would what is most suitable for your unique body is to have a deep core and pelvic floor assessment with a women's health physiotherapist who can guide you in your options.

HORMONAL CHANGES DURING PREGNANCY AND BEYOND

Other significant changes that take place during pregnancy and in lactating women are hormonal changes. The hormonal changes experienced during pregnancy and beyond are designed to support the growth of baby and the health of the mother. These hormonal changes also affect ligaments, cartilage, the nervous system, bone structure, and tendons.

There is much talk about the hormone relaxin and its effect on ligaments, causing them to become softer and stretchier during pregnancy. While this holds some truth, relaxin is not the only hormone that affects ligamentous changes during pregnancy. The key hormones that may affect ligaments during pregnancy and lactation are oestrogen, progesterone, testosterone, relaxin, sex hormone binding globulin, and insulin-like growth factor-1. The hormonal effects on ligaments during pregnancy serve to allow the pelvis to widen so that baby can pass through the birth canal but these hormonal changes affect all of the ligaments in our body, not just the pelvis. This is important because our ligaments are largely responsible for maintaining joint stability. The ligaments of the pelvic floor also play a particularly important role in providing support to the pelvic organs alongside the muscles of the pelvic floor. The additional 'give' of the ligaments of the pelvic floor is another reason for us to be mindful of our pelvic floor during pregnancy.

Relaxin is also commonly attributed to the increased ligament laxity that women experience in the postnatal period but relaxin levels are significantly reduced almost immediately after birth and are undetectable in the first few days postpartum. As mentioned earlier, lower oestrogen levels in lactating mothers are likely to be the main hormonal change that impacts pelvic health postpartum, and can increase symptoms of pelvic organ prolapse and incontinence. Oestrogen levels are usually normalised when the menstrual cycle returns.

PRESSURE ON THE PELVIC FLOOR

Lastly, there is increased pressure on the entire pelvic floor due to the weight of baby as well as the overall weight gained during pregnancy. Excessive weight gain during pregnancy increases the degree of stretch placed on the pelvic floor during pregnancy.

BIRTH RELATED BODY CHANGES

Multiple factors influence how your body is changed as a result of birth. Some physical changes that we experience during birth will improve over time, while other changes will have more lasting effects. Even when physical changes cannot be reversed, it doesn't mean that we are broken or that there is something wrong with us. Even when physical changes can be long-lasting, the practice of strengthening, nourishing, and connecting with our body will offer a significantly different experience compared to that which we would experience if we let ourselves be defined by the physical change.

Some of the factors that influence how our body is changed by giving birth are:

- Whether you have a vaginal or C-section delivery
- The duration of the second stage (or the pushing phase) of labour
- If any instruments were required
- If you had an episiotomy or tear - and the degree and direction of that tear
- The birth weight of the baby
- If you breastfeed, and for how long
- Your genetics
- Your age

When it comes to postnatal recovery and the impact of vaginal delivery compared to a C-section, I often hear women suggest that the recovery after C-section is a lot more challenging compared to the recovery of a vaginal delivery but it depends completely on the actual birth itself. There are many different ways a C-Section or a vaginal delivery can go, and without taking an individualised approach, there is no way we can assume that the recovery after one particular birth will be physically less challenging than another. If we consider the emotional, environmental, and energetic influences, the dynamic complexity of postpartum recovery becomes more apparent.

In this section, I will talk about the physical changes that occur as an impact of birth and particular interventions. However, we know that the impacts of birth are beyond the physical body. I feel it's important to affirm and recognise that every woman will have her own unique birth experience and creating assumptions as to how any woman may feel physically, emotionally, and energetically as a result of her birth experience, or making judgements around what would entail a more challenging recovery does not provide an accurate reflection of any woman's true experience. No one other than the woman herself can say or know what her experience *was like* and *is like* for her. Comparing women and their unique experience and casting any judgement is not helpful, nor would that judgement be accurate or true. We need to be careful what judgements or assumptions we pass onto others, and how we may compare our experience to someone else's. Your experience is yours to own. Every woman has the right to own her experiences, and it is our role as fellow women to support her in that.

Physically, a vaginal delivery will have more impact on the pelvic floor, compared to a C-Section delivery because most of the physical changes to the pelvic floor happen as the baby passes through the birth canal. On the other hand, a C-section delivery will have more impact on the abdominal wall as the incision passes through the muscles of the abdominal wall. This is not to say that no changes to the pelvic floor occur in the case of a C-section, because there are changes that occur during pregnancy. Likewise, women who birth vaginally will also have changes to the abdominal wall, like the separation that occurs at the Linea Alba that happens in pregnancy.

A second stage of labour that lasts longer than two hours is associated with increased pelvic floor changes. The use of forceps in delivery is associated with an increased risk of pelvic floor muscle avulsion (where the muscle is "torn away" from the bone), which results in an increased risk of anterior wall and uterine prolapse.

Perineal tears are generally graded on either a 4-point scale from a 1st degree tear to a 4th degree tear, or 6-point scale as described next.

Women who are told they had a 'perineal graze' have usually experienced a 1st degree tear.

- First-degree tear: Injury to perineal skin and/or vaginal mucosa
- Second-degree tear: Injury to perineum involving perineal muscles but not involving the anal sphincter
- Third-degree tear: Injury to perineum involving the anal sphincter complex
- Grade 3a tear: Less than 50% of external anal sphincter (EAS) thickness torn
- Grade 3b tear: More than 50% of EAS thickness torn
- Grade 3c tear: Both external anal sphincter and internal anal sphincter torn
- Fourth-degree tear: Injury to perineum involving the anal sphincter complex (external and internal anal sphincter) and anorectal mucosa

A 2nd degree tear affects both the vaginal skin and the perineal muscles – the superficial PF muscles - these tears will generally require sutures. 3rd and 4th degree tears require sutures and, according to the Royal College of Obstetricians and Gynaecologists Guidelines, should be offered by a skilled surgeon under anaesthetic. 3rd and 4th degree tears are the primary risk factor for faecal incontinence and are more prevalent after forceps delivery. (Royal College of Obstetricians and Gynecologists, 2015)

Larger birth weight babies are associated with increased changes to the pelvic floor. Genetics also play a role, and some women have a predisposition to a larger ratio of less dense collagen fibres, which creates more potential for stretching of the soft tissue fibres of the pelvic floor. Women who tend to get more stretch marks are likely to have this genetic predisposition. Age also plays its role, and the older we are the more likely we are to have changes to the deep core and pelvic floor as a result of pregnancy and birth.

In addition, numerous factors can influence overall deep core strength, coordination, endurance, and health including:

- Your overall level of fitness - while good overall fitness is beneficial to pelvic health, it is thought that there may be some levels of physical activity that may be harmful to pelvic health. We are yet to have strong evidence to guide women specifically regarding the impact of strenuous physical activity. (Nygaard et al, 2012: Majumdar et al 2013)
- Your bladder and bowel habits/health
- Chronic respiratory conditions and chronic constipation are also linked to an increased risk of developing pelvic floor changes and concerns
- The use of hormone replacement therapy
- How you allow yourself to recover and rebuild after birth
- How your deep core engages during movement, which can be affected by pregnancy birth, and musculoskeletal injury

CORE RESTORATION AND REBUILDING AFTER BIRTH

In general, women are exposed to very little education, information, and resources regarding rebuilding and recovery of the deep core and pelvic floor after birth. Though there has been a significant shift and improvement over the past decade, women are generally expected to seek out this information themselves. Depending on her unique circumstances, her environment, and the culture that surrounds her, some women will know that seeing a women's pelvic floor physiotherapist is one avenue of support that is available to her in her postpartum journey. Other women will have never even heard of their pelvic floor and know very little about the potential for pelvic health concerns to develop in the postnatal period, or if they already have pelvic concerns, they may not be aware that help exists.

One of the huge challenges with improving awareness and understanding of postnatal pelvic health, along with postnatal wellbeing in general, is that our experiences are so individual and unique, and our values are so personal, that creating overarching education that is beneficial to all women is very challenging. Some education models are aimed at inducing fear in women so that they don't overdo it in the early postnatal phase. The focus on potential risks becomes so intense that women are fraught with anxiety, and learn that their bodies are vulnerable and weak. Women are told things like, "Don't lift your children!" or that exercise is dangerous. These messages combined create enormous anxiety for women, leading them to feel like they are broken and incapable.

Other campaigns suggest that women are strong and, "We can do anything!" with images across social media of women running again and fitting into their jeans at six weeks postpartum. In instances like this, there is often no consideration for potential deep core and pelvic health concerns. Women who are exposed to these messages alone are at risk of being enticed into programs and regimes that focus on reaching certain goals and milestones, being drawn towards measuring themselves against other women, and unknowingly putting their bodies at potential risk of pelvic health concerns.

Other campaigns normalise the experience of incontinence and even laugh it off, which creates ongoing barriers for women to seek help and advice because they are led to believe that this is just how their body is now. Striking a balance between creating awareness

and understanding about postnatal deep core and pelvic floor recovery, while helping women to know that they are strong, resilient,
and capable is tricky. It requires a broad awareness, but with an individualised approach. I was running six weeks after my first baby,
comfortably with no incontinence and I never developed any sign of
pelvic organ prolapse. After my second birth, my recovery was very
different and it was many months before I was jogging with a sense
of assurance in my body. When some physiotherapists heard that I
was running again so early after my first pregnancy, they would say,
"She's going to prolapse", and I appreciated their concern, but it
wasn't the case. At the same time, having experienced such easy physical recovery after my first birth set me up with unrealistic expectations after my second birth. I could feel the difference in my body
and had I tried to run six weeks after my second birth, I think that I
probably would have caused a prolapse.

The complexity is amplified when we know that some women
can have significant pelvic changes, and have no symptoms. This is
why often therapists err on the side of caution when making recommendations to clients around movement and exercise. Furthermore,
what's important to one woman might be completely irrelevant to
another. If a therapist was to tell a runner not to run, she might feel
like her world is beginning to collapse around her, whereas if you
told a woman who doesn't enjoy high-intensity exercise not to run,
she probably wouldn't mind so much. But what if she was a mother
of three young children and you told her not to lift any of them? You
can imagine how she might feel.

For women who rely on particular movement and exercise for
emotional wellbeing, slowing things down and finding alternative
ways to move their bodies during the early postpartum period can be
challenging and frustrating. It's a common concern for new mothers that if they can't move their body in the ways that they love and

enjoy, and in ways that give them the emotional and energetic out-let that they require, that their mental health will spiral out of control. Risking particular pelvic health concerns may be their preferred option than knowing how trapped they will feel in their mind if they are not able to move in the way that gets their heart rate up and their body sweating like they are used to. I was one of these women! I know how this feels. But, there is also a deep opportunity here too for women to experience their body in a new way, and explore new ways of creating stillness and calm in their mind and body that doesn't require high intensity and high impact training. This is not to say that I support women being told to stop the movement that they love. I believe that it's important for us as human beings to move our bodies in ways that feel good. I believe that the therapist's role is to *show you how*, rather than to tell you that you can't. There is an opportunity for both approaches to exist in a way that strikes balance for us as individuals. What this means is that we need to find therapists that support us in our uniqueness as women; physically, emotionally, and spiritually. At the same time, we need to approach our journey with an open mind and a wide lens.

THE TRUTH ABOUT THE 6-WEEK CHECK

Many women are led to believe that if they have a six-week check by a doctor/midwife/ obstetrician/gynaecologist that they are 'safe' to return to exercise but the six-week check offered by your GP, obstetrician or midwife is very different from the one given by a women's health physiotherapist. Your GP/OB/midwife is usually assessing for postnatal complications such as infection, retained placenta, suspicious ongoing bleeding, or other medical complications. While this is important, and while it might not be considered safe to return to exercise if you were to have some kind of medical complication, the absence of any of these concerning cases has nothing to do with what exercises may be considered safe in relation to deep core and pelvic floor health.

A postnatal check conducted by a women's health physiotherapist is very different from that conducted by any of the previously mentioned healthcare providers. A good pelvic floor physio will assess:

- The pelvic floor muscles for strength, coordination, and endurance
- The integrity of the pelvic floor as a whole
- The presence of POP and the perceived risk of developing POP
- Abdominal separation and the tensile strength of the Linea Alba
- How the muscles of the deep core activate during movement

They should also be able to provide personalised guidance for recovery and advice regarding returning to a particular movement and activity including work, exercise, and guidance around sexual activity.

RETURNING TO EXERCISE AFTER BIRTH

One of the biggest challenges women face after birth is returning to movement and exercise. The fact that our lifestyle changes dramatically with a newborn, and we have the challenges of fitting it all in, as well as the fact that our sleep routines have changed, and we have the physical demands of nurturing a new life are all reasons why returning to movement and exercise can be challenging. From my experience though, the bigger challenge for new mothers when it comes to returning to movement and exercise is getting to know, re-connect with, and build a positive relationship with their body after birth.

During pregnancy and after birth our bodies change dramatically in a short time. Add to that the new demands of being a mother, whether it be for the first time or not, and we have a lot to navigate amongst what can seem like a whirlwind of change. While it is help-ful to know a general progression of exercise, and how to monitor and modify your movement using the ABCDE technique (p. 172 - 181), I believe none of this will matter so much if you don't give yourself the chance to connect with your body and create the foun-dations for a positive relationship with your body after birth. Not taking the time to reconnect with and rebuild our bodies after birth can leave us feeling weak, like our body is failing us, frustrated with our slow progress, disappointed and exhausted.

Although I've offered some time frames in the guidelines that fol-low, it's important to know that these time frames are based on un-complicated births, and that every woman will have her unique path. These time frames are not goals that you need to meet, but they offer some information as to what a gradual progression of exercise and movement can look like. The most important thing is that you listen to your body without creating expectations of where you should be by a certain point in time.

In the first six weeks after baby is born, the most important thing to focus on is rest, recovery, and nurturing your needs as a mother and as a woman. Taking time to physically lie down and let the mus-cles of the deep core and pelvic floor rest from the demands of your day and gravity is helpful for these muscles' recovery.

There is some anecdotal evidence to support the use of com-pressive garments to offer additional support to the abdominal wall. During the first six weeks, you may like to commence the chin tucks described in the DRAM recovery section (p. 189-198) of this book. Additionally, pelvic floor exercises and deep core awareness practices are safe and helpful. If you have had a C-section, scar management as described later on in this book can be commenced when it has healed sufficiently. Use the guidance of your health care provider to know when you can begin scar massage and management. Similarly, if you had an episiotomy or tear to the perineal tissue, you may like to start with some gentle massage to this area to stimulate healthy recovery. Again, use the advice of your health care provider for when this will be safe to commence. Perineal massage techniques are described further on.

In terms of movement and exercise at 0-6 weeks postpartum, the following is recommended:

- Gentle walking
- Core awareness exercises
- Pelvic floor exercise with a focus on relaxation as well as gentle strength/co-ordination/endurance exercises

At about six weeks postnatal, it is recommended that you seek advice from a pelvic floor therapist. You can choose to see them earlier if you wish, but generally, there is a lot of early recovery occurring at this time and the information you receive could be quite limited. A vaginal pelvic floor assessment will give you more accurate and individualised advice. The early recovery recommendations such as the chin tucks and perineal massage can be continued. In addition, you may like to consider the following exercise options:

- Low impact aerobics – preferably with a postnatal specialist
- Postnatal classes including modified circuit style/lightweight training, Pilates, or yoga

- Aqua programs including modified aqua aerobics or swimming (once bleeding has ceased and you are cleared of any signs of infection)

It is generally recommended that you avoid high-impact exercise (such as running and jumping) for at least three (3) months postpartum. From three months onward you may like to introduce modified impact training using a progressive training approach and gradually increase intensity, impact and weight training, remembering not to ignore any signs of deep core imbalance or pelvic stress such as incontinence or pelvic heaviness. Using the ABCDE approach will help guide your graduated return to exercise.

EXERCISES TO AVOID IN THE EARLY POSTPARTUM PERIOD (0-3 MONTHS)

Here are some exercises that I recommend avoiding in the early postnatal period. This is not an exhaustive list, but it will give you an idea of what exercises have greater risks of significantly increasing intra-abdominal pressure and therefore developing pelvic floor symptoms.

- Abdominal exercises such as sit-ups and crunches
- Weighted abdominal exercises
- Exercises with both feet off the ground such as a V-sit, boat pose, Pilates hundreds, double-leg lowers
- Full plank position on hands and feet (e.g. hovers, plank holds, push-ups)
- Deep lunges, wide side lunges, wide-legged squats
- Jumping
- Heavy lifting

• Any exercise where you feel direct downward pressure on the pelvic floor

C-SECTION SCAR MANAGEMENT

For general comfort, as well as deep core health it's important that the tissues around your C-section incision site heal well. Good scar management helps to ensure that the soft tissue around the incision site heals in such a way that this tissue is pliable and moveable. This helps the muscles of the abdominal wall to glide and slide across one another. Massage also helps to increase sensation and stimulate blood flow for healing.

Scar management can be commenced as soon as your incision site has healed well enough. Use the guidance of your health care provider to know when scar management is safe to begin. If you have had your C-section a long time ago and didn't use any of the techniques described here, you can begin to use them at any time. While it may not have the same impact as early intervention would have, they are still safe and offer a nice way to reconnect with this part of your body in a new and nurturing way.

Some women feel very uneasy touching their scar for a number of different reasons. It may be a reminder of the birth trauma they experienced, some dislike the appearance of the scar, and others are simply unsure if they should be touching it or not. If you do feel quite uneasy touching your scar, taking a graduated approach may be helpful. Begin with simply resting your hands on your scar and breathing into the space. Let your whole body relax as you do this. You may like to then progress to a generalised abdominal massage, using the techniques described in the Womb Massage practice (p. 281 - 284). When you feel ready and comfortable, begin incorporating the specific scar massage techniques described below.

I generally suggest using coconut oil, caster oil, or any natural based oil/lotion for scar massage. In the early days, a non-fragranced oil/lotion is preferred. Using two fingers, gently massage over the scar line with the same pressure you would use if you were patting a cat.

Moving in three directions is recommended:

- Across the scar line to the left and right
- Up and down over the scar line
- Small circles across the scar line

If you find an area that feels particularly ropey or sticky concentrate on that area for a little longer. You can perform your massage as often as you like. Even if you do feel very comfortable touching your scar incorporating this style of massage into a Womb Massage can help to build your relationship with your body.

PERINEAL MASSAGE

Again, some women may feel quite hesitant to massage this area after a tear or episiotomy. Ask for guidance from your health care provider for when you may commence scar massage. This will generally be when sutures have dissolved and healthy scar tissue has started to form.

Comfortable positions for perineal massage are:

- In a reclined sitting position with the knees bent and spread wide with pillows to support you
- In side lie - with the knees bent, and approaching with your hand from behind

• Standing with one leg supported on a chair

Begin with simply breathing into the pelvic bowl, directing your breath to the perineal space. You may feel a gentle stretching sensation when you do so. Using one or two fingers, gently massage over the skin that sits between the vagina and the anus. Small circular motions, and sweeping motions forwards and backward in all directions generally feel good. Next place your thumb at the entrance of the vagina, and with gentle pressure create sweeping motions in a half-moon direction focusing on the tissue on the posterior aspect of the vagina that sits between the anus and the vagina, as well as the tissue to the left and right. Often women find using the right hand to massage the left half of the perineal tissue vaginally and the right hand to massage the left perineal tissue comfortable. If you find an area that feels particularly ropey or tender you can choose to focus your massage there. Use gentle pressure, this should be comfortable and never painful.

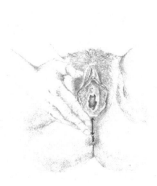

PERINEAL SCAR MASSAGE

PERINEAL SCAR MASSAGE

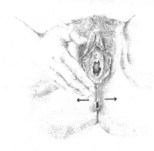

PERINEAL SCAR MASSAGE

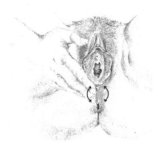

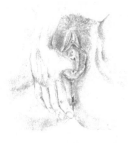

INTERNAL PERINEAL SCAR MASSAGE

BIRTH RECOVERY

DEFINING THE POSTNATAL PERIOD

Defining the postnatal period is challenging as there is no real consensus as to what is considered postnatal, both from a medical standpoint and a societal standpoint. Because there is a lot of emphasis on 'The 6 Week Postnatal Check-up' many women are led to believe that their postnatal recovery is just six weeks in length but there is increasing acceptance and awareness that there are continuing significant physiological and biological changes occurring during the fourth trimester, generally thought to be the first three months postpartum. I love our increasing awareness of the postnatal phase and the fact that postpartum recovery takes much longer than the six weeks that modern society may have us believe. The 'fourth trimester' as a term for a recognised phase is valuable for women. It helps us to recognise that postnatal recovery continues to occur beyond the first six weeks postpartum, and it encourages us to focus on taking care of ourselves as mothers in this early postnatal phase.

With our world being so connected, the fourth trimester is becoming something that more and more women appreciate and acknowledge. It's becoming part of our normal societal language, though perhaps more prominent in some circles than others.

The concern I have with the phrase the 'fourth trimester' is that it *may* cause some women to believe that they should feel a particular way after a particular period after birth, in this case three months postpartum. I don't want to devalue this recognition of this precious time of recovery and self-connection, I simply want to recognise that there is no time frame for when we may feel normal again after birth. There is a continued gradual restoration phase that is more subtle that, from my experience working with mothers, continues for about two years postpartum. We are never the same once we have given birth, and even women who recognise that still sense that something shifts within them after a period after birth where they begin to feel 'normal' again in their body after birth. We cannot rush this process, and the more we place expectations on ourselves to feel a particular way by a certain time, the more likely we are to feel disconnected, disappointed and uneasy in our body. Letting go of the time frames and letting your body lead and reveal your pathway feels so much more freeing, pleasant and peaceful.

Because of the unique physical, emotional and energetic nature of the postpartum period, it is important that we recognise how a woman in this phase is different to women who have either never had children, or who have had children many years ago and are now experiencing new transition phases in their life, such as perimenopause and menopause. Our postnatal journey and transition into motherhood is dynamic and complex. Some schools of thought maintain that once a woman has birthed, she will always be postnatal. This has value and validity to it because even women who have birthed and are now moving through new transition phases, such as menopause for example, will have very different experiences in their body and their life compared to women who haven't. However, a woman who has had a baby more recently, say three months ago versus three years ago, will have very different challenges and needs.

Continued research is required into so many topics that pertain to the unique nature of women's bodies, including the postnatal period and our transition into motherhood. I believe continued research into these topics along with a deep appreciation for the transition phases that women go through in their lifetime, new language, ideas and ways of being will develop that highlight and recognise this continued transitioning.

POSTNATAL RECOVERY – A JOURNEY NOT A DESTINATION

When we talk about 'postnatal recovery' I think it's important to consider and understand what the phrase recovery means. Recovery is sometimes understood as a point to get to, a destination and we think, "When I've recovered I will feel good". Accepting this understanding of the term 'recovery' could lead us to believe that we can only feel good once we have recovered after birth. The mindset then focuses on working towards a point in time in the future, and we're left waiting to feel good. This mindset takes us out of body presence and leads us to continue to practice the striving that many of us have become accustomed to. If we consider the term recovery as a journey, we can sense that feeling good now is available to us. We don't need to wait until some point in the future when our bodies are different, instead, we can sense the beauty and the joy now. This simple act of embracing body presence and honouring the journey invites a new level of permission for us to accept and meet ourselves where we are with more kindness and self-compassion.

YOUR BIRTH/ABORTION/MISCARRIAGE
EXPERIENCE MATTERS

We recognise time and time again that usually after we give birth, our focus goes to the baby. We often talk about how little time we dedicate to nurturing the mother and I think we are getting somewhat better at recognising how much energetic nourishment is required for the mother in order to be able to then nourish a family. I feel though that if we don't take some time to acknowledge and process our birth experience energetically and emotionally (particularly in the case of birth trauma), we continue to move through our life feeling broken.

Often, it's not until a woman is sitting in front of me recounting her birth experience, usually in a quite matter of fact way, and I ask her, "How did you *feel* about your birth experience?" that a woman gives herself the time to actually reflect on how she felt and still feels about her birth. Tears well up, and she has a moment of confusion before saying, "I didn't even know that that's how I felt about it all."

Many women think that their emotions around their birth experience are not valid. "I know I have a healthy baby, and compared to other women my experience is nothing, so I shouldn't be complaining..." This is often the same for women who have experienced miscarriage or abortion. We nullify our experiences. "I had a choice, and I made it, so I need to deal with it and get on with my life." Yes, you had a choice, a hard and difficult one, and just because you made a particular decision, it doesn't mean that grief, loss, deep sadness, and pain are not part of your experience. You are not wrong to feel these things. You deserve to have your pain met without judgement. You deserve to have the time and space to heal. Be where you are, feel how you feel.

"It was an early miscarriage. I was only seven weeks, so it doesn't count." It counts. You count and your experience matters. There is no marker that will indicate how you experience your loss, like seven weeks is less painful than 10. Your pain is your pain, and you don't need to pretend like it doesn't exist to make others feel comfortable. Your pain desires and deserves to be expressed, not suppressed.

Your feelings around your birth experience are valid. Comparison to another woman's experience is not required. Trying to diminish, wrong, or abolish your feelings doesn't help them to go away. Dealing with emotions in this way helps them to continue to live inside of us, to grow, and to make us feel like victims of our experience. Recognising your feelings, acknowledging them, and allowing time to simply sit with the emotion without trying to change them is what helps us to process our feelings. When we feel our feelings, we are no longer hostage to them, but rather a witness to them. When we can witness our feelings, we can begin to feel free and more at peace. Finding or creating safe spaces to give voice to our emotions, to be present in our body, and to feel seen, heard, and witnessed is powerful. Seek your safe space. Let your voice be heard.

THE NATURAL BIRTH MOVEMENT

The natural birth movement, sometimes called the empowered birth movement, has some great benefits like helping women feel less afraid of birth, trusting more in our body's ability to birth, and knowing we have a say and a choice in how we birth. Yes to all of that! But there is an ugly beast that was born with the natural birth movement, the one that wrongs women who require medical intervention. "Oh, she must have had some kind of energetic block!" or "Oh, she got too much up in her head, and wasn't in her body enough." She did x, y, or z wrong. NO! The whole purpose of this movement is to support women. Somehow it so often ends up blaming women, their choices, and their circumstances that were beyond their control. You are NO less a woman if you require or required or chose to have some type of birth intervention. Don't ever let anyone tell you otherwise!

"BREAST IS BEST"... UNTIL IT'S NOT

Breast is best! What a catchy title for a very important evidence-based educational message. Again, however, the judgement experienced by women who are unable to breastfeed is horrendous. Breastfeeding takes effort, patience, and sometimes it's freaking painful. Sure, I encourage women to persevere, because it is challenging. But sometimes breast isn't best, and women who have made this very challenging decision not to continue with breastfeeding don't need anyone's judgement. That's one problem with this campaign. Just like so many others, it riddles women with guilt and shame because they feel like they can't live up to the expectations, they feel like their body has failed, they feel like less of a woman or that they aren't a 'real woman'. This is not helpful in any way. If we are concerned for what is best for baby, we would understand that creating environments where mothers feel supported and can sense their wholeness is far more important than how a mother feeds their baby.

WHAT PREGNANCY, BIRTH, & MOTHERHOOD TEACHES US

Just as Menarche is our initiation into womanhood and a beautiful introduction to our cyclical nature as women, pregnancy offers us an opportunity to see more fully how we relate to our body as a whole. The rapid changes that occur in our body during pregnancy can be very confronting. How we feel about these changes reveals to us how we see our body. Personally, I felt quite inconvenienced by the changes in my body during my first two pregnancies, because I viewed my body as a functional machine, and judged it harshly on how it looked. By my third pregnancy, I had done much of the inner work that allowed me to embrace the changes that were happening. Even though I was less active in my pregnancy compared to previous pregnancies, I didn't criticise myself for being lazy or less capable, I simply saw my body as different now to how it once was. I know that if I hadn't learned a more Body Conscious way of connecting to myself that I would have had a much more strained relationship with my body and it's changing function.

During pregnancy, we can also be looking towards motherhood an imagining the type of mother we envision ourselves to be. Whilst there is nothing wrong with this, there becomes a question of how far ahead we look into the future trying to control and predict how we will be and act, rather than being led by life itself in the moment.

On a more energetic and spiritual level pregnancy is a time where we can reflect on our creative power. We can sense our body bringing a soul from the realm of greater consciousness into our physical world. We can use this opportunity to contemplate how ease filled our body does this. We don't need to think up the steps, or take any form of particular action. Our body is simply in the process of creation. All we need to do is nurture ourselves in a way that feels good to nurture the growth of this little human.

Pregnancy offers a beautiful parallel for all forms of creativity and how we birth an inspired idea into reality. Creativity isn't reliant on constant action, or thinking up steps. Contemplating pregnancy reflects the power of allowing, rest, and gradual growth without force.

Following are some questions for reflection regarding pregnancy and your relationship with your body during pregnancy.

If you are currently pregnant, you can contemplate these questions as you feel today. If you are postpartum, you may like to explore how you related to your body during pregnancy.

- How do I feel about my body?
- In particular, how do I feel about the changes in my body?
- What changes do I feel inconvenienced by? Ashamed of?
- How does this reflect my overall relationship with my body?
- How could I be kinder and more patient with my body?
- If I were to embrace the changes in my body during this transition, what would I do more of? What would I stop doing?
- How can I allow myself to create in a way that is reflective of my natural rhythm and flow?
- Where can I stop forcing, and instead simply allow?
- If I were to approach the changes in my body with a deep sense of self-love, self-kindness, and self-connection - how would that look/feel?
- How am I nurturing my whole self (mind, body, soul) during my pregnancy?
- When I consider how my body is creating life, where does that take me?

Birth is a profound teacher. It will teach us everything from how we trust our body, what we value, how we allow others to influence our decisions, where we hand over our personal power, to how we feel voicing our truth and honouring our autonomy. Birth teaches us the delicate dance between our creative potential and our ability to create based on our personal choices, and what is beyond our control and in the hands of the universe.

If you are approaching birth, you may like to consider the following questions for reflection:

- What stories do I have about birth?
- Are these stories mine?
- What stories about birth do I want to let go of?
- If I was to approach my birth with a sense of trust in my self and my body, what would that look like/feel like?
- What has me feel safe and supported in my birth journey?

If you are postpartum, you may like to reflect on these questions:

- How do I feel about my birth?
- If I was to support myself moving through my birth experience, who/what would I call into my energetic space?
- What did my birth/s teach me? What wisdom did I receive?
- Where have I shared my birth story/stories?
- How would I like to move through my birth experience?
- What would have me feel safe and supported to do that?
- What do I choose for myself now?

Motherhood brings a beautiful opportunity to witness ourselves in dynamic relationship with another human being. Motherhood shows us how we balance our own needs with the needs of another human. Motherhood tends to be a time in our life where we question everything, creating an opportunity for us to live in more alignment to our self. If we take the time to reflect, we can start to see more clearly how we may be living in a way that is defined by stories we have learned and narratives we have created around what is possible in our lives and what is possible as a mother. We are stripped back to our core. We are shown all of the ways in which we had created an identify for ourselves. We are gifted an opportunity to recreate ourselves, shedding all of the things that no longer serve.

Motherhood reflective questions:

- What are my biggest challenges in motherhood right now?
- What are they offering me? What are they teaching me?
- How do I give back to my self as a mother?
- How could I be more gentle/kind to myself as a mother?
- What does my mothering 'rhythm' feel like?
- How would I like my mothering rhythm to feel?
- If I was to embrace MY mothering rhythm - what would I do? What would I stop doing?
- Where are the lines of separation between me as a mother and me as a whole woman?
- If I was to integrate motherhood into my whole life more, how would that look? How would that feel?
- What personal values is motherhood highlighting for me?
- Where do I feel limited by the fact that I am a mother? Is this really true for me? If I could create another more meaningful narrative around this, what would it be?

6

SEX AND SENSUALITY

When I talk with women about how they would like to feel in relationship to sex, three things commonly come up:

- They would like to have a healthy interest in sex.
- They would like to feel embodied, and able to be present in their body during sex, rather than concerning themselves with how they might appear or how they are 'performing', and;
- They would like to enjoy pleasurable and satisfying sex.

I invite you to take some time to consider how you would like to experience sex and how you would like to feel in relationship to sex.

When we consider the commonalities regarding how women want to feel during sex, we can understand what is required in our relationship with our self our body, and our chosen partner/s to have the type of experience we desire.

To have a healthy interest in sex, to be able to feel embodied, and to enjoy pleasurable and satisfying sex we need:

- Positive pelvic health and healthy hormones
- Ample energy and vitality
- A positive association with sex and pleasure
- To feel safe and respected
- For sex to feel comfortable and pleasurable, and not painful
- To have a positive relationship with our body including our feminine body
- To be able to communicate our needs and desires
- A willingness to be vulnerable, curious, and open

For many women, in addition to the above, they also desire:

- A deep sense of love and spiritual connection

Much of what I've already talked about in this book, and the practices that create positive body connection and pelvic health, are principles and practices that can have a positive influence on our sexual desire, connection, and experience. In the following section, I invite you to explore in more detail your relationship to sex, your experience of sex, and how you would like sex to feel. The information that I share is designed to be part of a whole-body integrated approach to your wellness. While I will talk briefly about hormones and feeling safe in your body during sex, I acknowledge that some women will require support that goes beyond the scope of this book. If you sense this is you, I encourage you to seek the appropriate assistance for you.

SENSUAL AND SEXUAL ENERGY

Before we continue talking about sex, I want to share with you how I differentiate sensual energy and sexual energy. The two are intimately related and I believe that a positive sensual self-connection underpins a positive sexual connection and therefore a more positive relationship with, and experience of sex. Sensual energy to me has a simmering, bubbling, more continuous energy compared to sexual energy. Sexual energy, to me, has more of an energy that continually increases to a more explosive point where it then declines and almost meets the foundational sensual energy. When we are in relationship with a partner, nurturing both the sensual energetic relationship along with the sexual energetic relationship is essential for enjoying a positive connection. For us to be present in our body during sex and to enjoy the full experience and pleasure of sex, I also believe that we need to nurture our own sensual self-connection. What this looks like for each of us will be unique to us.

In my relationship with myself, I connect to sensual energy through things like movement, warm baths, being in and observing nature, and through the simple act of taking short pauses throughout my day to become more mindful of my experiences, like stopping to sip a cup of tea and taking the time to smell it, taste it and feel its warmth throughout my body.

In my relationship with my husband, sensual connection is created by listening more intently, being playful in our interactions so that we don't slip into the mundane day-to-day interactions without appreciating one another, taking moments of gratitude when I witness his presence with our children, and as cheesy as it sounds taking moments to simply look at his face and admire his features.

For me, sensual connection to self or another human being is about connecting to the experience of pleasure and joy.

Perhaps you may like to consider what does sensuality and sensual energy look/feel like to you? What does sexual energy look and feel like to you?

SENSUAL AND SEXUAL
SELF-CONNECTION REFLECTION

Here are some questions to contemplate and perhaps journal about:

- Do I take time to connect to myself sensually?
- What does that look like for me?
- How do I feel when I connect with myself in this way?
- How does that change my experience of life?
- How does that change my experience of sex?
- Have I explored my own body and self-pleasure?

- What are my thoughts around self-pleasure and masturbation?
- What does sensual energy look like & feel like to me?
- How am I expressing myself sensually?
- What brings me pleasure & joy in my life?
- Where in my life would I like to explore a deeper sense of sensual connection? What would that look like?
- What is my relationship to pleasure? What is my relationship to receiving pleasure? How does self-pleasure feel?
- If I was to connect more deeply to my sensual energy, what would I do more of?
- If I was to connect more deeply with my sensual energy, what would I stop doing?

EXPLORING YOUR BELIEFS ABOUT SEX

We live in a society that encourages women to spend so much time, money and effort on trying to be 'sexy'. But what happens in the moment when you start to feel sexy?

For some of us, we immediately feel disgusted with ourselves; dirty and gross. Others feel like they become 'too much', too comfortable in her own skin and too confident. It's a lose/lose situation. Not sexy enough, or too sexy.

Depending on the kind of culture you grew up in, sex might be seen as a dirty act and something to be ashamed of. Sex could be a purely functional act done for the purpose of procreation only, not for the pleasure and powerful connections that can be experienced. On the other hand, it could be a way to validate a woman's worth – if she has a lot of sex, she is popular and attractive.

By bringing our awareness to the conflicting messages we are exposed to in regards to sex, and by bringing our awareness to our own beliefs around sex, we can start to notice where our thoughts and beliefs about sex might not feel true for us. Once we recognise what beliefs don't feel true, we can create new beliefs, new habits and new choices around how we approach and view sex.

Here are some questions to contemplate your beliefs around sex. They can give you some new insight into your ideas and inspire contemplation towards how you may like to shift perspectives to change your experience of sex. The suggestions under each question are not designed to be answers that you need to choose from, but rather are offered to stimulate your thoughts.

What is it that you want to experience or feel during sex?

- Body present/embodied
- Pleasure
- Connection to self and partner
- Fully expressed
- Safe
- Being more of yourself

What do you believe is the purpose of sex?

- Pleasure - for both you and your partner
- Creating connection – physical and emotional
- Expression of love
- Co-creating and procreation creating new life

What meaning do you attach to **not** wanting to have sex?

- I am unwilling to connect with my partner
- It's a normal and healthy part of my nature

- I am not pleasing my partner
- I have healthy boundaries
- It's simply part of my cyclical nature

What do you believe about sex?

- It's dirty and shameful
- It's an expression of love and an opportunity to create connection
- I need to please my partner
- My needs and desires are unimportant

Where do your beliefs about sex come from?

- My parents/teachers/family/other influential people growing up
- My religious/cultural background
- Friends
- Past relationships/sexual experiences
- The media

Do these beliefs feel truly aligned for you?

How do these beliefs serve you and impact your experience of sex?

If you could believe anything about sex, what would it be?

How does sex feel to you?

INTIMACY DOESN'T HAVE TO LEAD TO SEX

Do you ever avoid being intimate with your partner because you think that if you start something you have to go all the way? I know that I used to avoid having playful or romantic moments with my partner because I believed if I did, he would automatically think we were going to have sex. In reality, all it took was for me to initiate one vulnerable conversation where I told him the story that I had created in my mind, where my husband offered reassurance that this wasn't the case.

We can attach so much emphasis to the *outcome* of a particular interaction, and create particular scenarios in our mind that stop us from having the spontaneous, playful, romantic, and sensual interactions that may or may not lead to sex. When we only allow ourselves to have them when we want the interaction to lead to sex, it reinforces our belief that we can only engage with our partner in this way when we want it to result in sex. This also leads us to reinforce the emphasis being on the outcome of having sex – the orgasm, which can take us away from being present to the entire experience.

STAYING IN YOUR BODY DURING
SEX AND INTIMACY

How present in your body are you during intimacy and sex? Many women recognise that they can be very much in their heads; thinking about their next move, imagining what their partner is thinking, wondering what they look like, or trying to hide how they look. Sometimes we aren't even thinking about the sex we are having, but instead caught up in our heads with our to-do list. Some women recognise that they consciously disconnect from their body during moments of sex and intimacy because being present in their body feels so uncomfortable or unsafe.

Becoming more present in our body during sex can be challenging because of its highly vulnerable nature. Practicing body presence in less vulnerable circumstances, where we have the spaciousness to explore our body while feeling completely safe can help us to begin practicing body presence, which can then lead to becoming more embodied during sex. Finding opportunities in your day-to-day life to *simply be* in your body is a great, accessible, and easy place to start. Creating the intention to simply become more aware of when you tend to get in your head, and creating opportunities that bring you back into your body through simple practices can be powerful. Many of the practices in this book focus on body presence and by embodying these practices you will become more able to maintain body presence.

As you become more familiar with practicing body presence in non-sexual ways, you may then like to invite yourself to practice becoming more body present during sexual self-pleasure and then integrate this experience into sex and intimacy with your partner. In this way, you are inviting a progressive practice of being body present beginning with practices that may feel more accessible and less vulnerable.

RECOGNISING THE IMPACT OF TRAUMA

When contemplating your ability and willingness to be body-present during sex, it's important to contemplate how safe you feel being in your body at other times. Sometimes we don't recognise how our experiences can shape how we experience our body during sex, particularly in the instance of non-sexual feminine trauma including birth trauma, medical trauma, and surgical trauma. Women who have experienced these kinds of trauma often find it challenging to be present in their body during sex and have a diminished interest in sex. When women don't have the awareness of the potential impact of such experiences, they often begin blaming themselves and their body for not having a desire for sex and may also feel confused as to why they have such a disinterest or a sense of being absent from their body during sex. The simple acknowledgement of how trauma can influence our experience of simply feeling safe to be in our body, can open a pathway for healing to begin. In healing from trauma, a newfound interest in sex, along with a more in body experience of sex, can grow.

KNOWING YOUR FEMININE BODY SEXUALLY

Earlier in this book, I've talked about why it's important to understand your feminine body from an all-encompassing health perspective. One big reason to understand your feminine body is so that you can enjoy sexual pleasure. I think it's important that we get to know our feminine body both from an anatomical and physiological perspective, as well as more intimately in a way that we can appreciate our body as a sacred space and enjoy the pleasure that it has to offer. Getting to know your body intimately requires us to move through the barrier of shame that is present for many of us. This may be shame around receiving pleasure in general and, in particular, shame related to personal pleasure and masturbation. So many women don't engage in personal pleasure because they feel embarrassed about doing so. The guilt attached to self-stimulation can be so profound that it takes away any of the pleasure that would possibly be enjoyed.

Becoming curious about the stories that you tell yourself about self-pleasure, or what you think and feel about self-pleasure and why you might think/feel that is a great place to focus your awareness if you shy away from it.

The practice then becomes exploring your feminine body in ways that bring you pleasure and joy and that help you move through those shame barriers. It may begin with exploring your body in a non-sexual way and finding ways to access pleasure in ways that feel comfortable and safe. Any of the Body Connection Practices in this book are designed to help you find pleasure in your body, in particular the Womb Massage, Getting to Know Your Feminine Body, movement for joy and pleasure, and self-directed Pelvic Massage will help you explore your feminine body in a way that feels safe because you are in control.

Extending the practice to include sexual pleasure may feel uncomfortable at first. Remember that focusing on a particular outcome may distance you from remaining present in your body. Rather than focusing on reaching orgasm, focus on the sensations that you feel in your body.

Creating an affirmation that resonates with you may help you to move through any shame you may feel. Some suggestions are:

- I deserve to feel pleasure in my body.
- It is safe to feel pleasure in my body.
- My body is designed to enjoy pleasure.
- It is natural to feel pleasure in my body.

I firmly believe that affirmations only help if they resonate and feel true for you at some level. As you reprogram your mindset to connect with self-pleasure that is not linked to shame, you will become to feel more confident and sense more truth in your affirmation, and at some point. will no longer require it.

Remaining with your breath and staying connected to the sensations that you feel in your body helps you stay present in your body without becoming distracted by stories that your mind may create.

SEX SHOULD NOT BE PAINFUL

Many women that experience pain with sex accept it as normal. Sex should be pleasurable and enjoyable, *not painful*. If you experience pain with sex, the first step towards enjoying more pleasurable sex is to recognise that you don't need to put up with it and that pathways to enjoying pain fee sex are available to you.

Like with many pain experiences in our body, pain with sex is multifaceted and layered. Understanding that there is probably a physical contribution to your pain, as well as a likely energetic and emotional contribution too can help to take a more holistic approach to healing your pain. Even when pain starts purely as a physical symptom from physical causes, over time this has emotional and energetic impacts.

Often pain with sex is a result of pelvic tension. The pelvic tension can sometimes be the original cause of the pain. Other times pelvic tension may be secondary to the actual cause of the pain. Over time the body learns to anticipate the pain, causing the pelvic floor to contract in anticipation, which has a spiral effect leading to ongoing pain with sex, and in some cases pelvic pain in general. Some of the common things women with an overactive or hypervigilant pelvic floor say they experience during sex are:

- Feeling unable to relax, even though they want to
- Pain with penetrative sex
- A male partner saying, "It feels like you don't want me to enter," or something along the lines of, "It feels like you're pushing me out".
- A sensation of feeling tense in the pelvic floor

In the case where there has been emotional/energetic trauma, women often experience:

- A feeling of being unable to be present in their body during sex
- A sensation of leaving their body during sex
- A disconnect from their pelvic space, not only during sex, but always

The experience of pain during sex is traumatic in itself so when women experience pain during sex, they can develop a feeling of being unable to be present in their body and a disconnection from their pelvic space. To experience pain-free, pleasurable sex, a holistic integrated approach that considers the physical attributes of your pain in conjunction with the energetic, emotional, environmental, and spiritual aspects is required.

If you experience pain with sex, considering the following questions may help you to understand some of the possible contributing factors to your pain. They may also invite a different and gentle curiosity that explores how you may relieve the physical factors that contribute to your pain.

- When did you first experience pain with sex?
- Have you always experienced pain with sex or is this something new?
- If it is something new, what has changed? Have you had a life transition? Perhaps given birth? Changed partners? Moved through menopause? Experienced a traumatic event?
- Do you experience pain with sex every time? Or is it just sometimes?

- Is there a pattern to your pain? Perhaps you recognise that your pain seems to align with your menstrual cycle, or maybe is increased during times that you feel stressed?
- Do you experience pain in all positions, or only in particular positions?
- Do you experience pain with penetration at the entrance of the vagina? Or does it feel more like a deep thudding?

The timing of when your pain began can be a good indicator of what may have triggered the initial onset of the discomfort. If you have moved through a life transition, the nature of that transition can give you some insight as to how you may like to approach your healing. If you can identify a life experience or transition that seemed to be the beginning of your pain, I invite you to contemplate not only the physiological changes that may have occurred in your body, but also how you felt emotionally and energetically at this time and how you have supported yourself since then to express and work with that emotion/energy?

For example, if there has been a significant hormonal change, like menopause, or if you are breastfeeding, where oestrogen levels are decreased and may result in vaginal dryness, you may like to explore different options for improving vaginal lubrication such as a water-based lubricant, or dietary changes to help stimulate oestrogen production. A stressful life event may have triggered the onset of pain. We often don't realise it, but many women hold their stress in their pelvic region causing pelvic tension. This increase in tension can be enough to stimulate pain with intercourse. In this case, creating lifestyle changes that help to reduce stress, and focusing on relaxing the muscles of the deep core and pelvic floor will be helpful. Determining the root cause of your pain can help guide your pathway to enjoyable pain-free sex.

Sometimes pain with penetration can indicate overactivity of the muscles of the pelvic floor, whereas a deep thudding sensation can be more indicative of uterine decent. Sometimes certain positions feel more comfortable because you are in control of the depth and pace of penetration. If you would like to enjoy more variety in your sex, but feel like certain positions are restricted due to pain, perhaps you would like to open more dialogue with your partner to offer some direction of what feels good in terms of depth and pace of penetration. Some helpful questions may be:

- Does the pain get better with time during sex?
- Do you feel rushed into sex? Are you focusing on orgasm, rather than the entire experience?
- Do you have sex to 'please' your partner, even when you don't feel like it?

If the pain improves with time, perhaps you sense your body simply needs more time to become aroused before penetrative sex. Some women who experience pain with sex say that they anticipate the pain, so rather than enjoying foreplay they have a sense of urgency to get it over and done with. Some women say that sex has become more about pleasing their partner, rather than enjoying the sex for themselves or as a couple. This happens even in instances where women feel that they have a partner who is very understanding and open. In this situation, I feel it's important that women connect to, and honour, their own needs in the same way that they consider their partner's needs.

In the following pages, I offer some thoughts around how you can begin to honour your needs and desires for pleasure.

TARYN GAUDIN

WHAT FEELS GOOD TODAY MIGHT
NOT FEEL GOOD TOMORROW

As women, our bodies have a very evident cyclical nature and rhythm. Our hormonal fluctuations mean that our body's sensitivity and our likes and dislikes change throughout the different phases of our cycle. Things like breast sensitivity and our natural vaginal lubrication change across our cycle, which means that the subtleties of what we like and dislike during intercourse can also change. Sometimes you might enjoy intense pressure around the nipple, other times that would feel uncomfortable, perhaps even painful. We aren't necessarily consistent with what we like/dislike, because we are fluid beings.

Sitting by the fire recently, my husband and I were talking about exactly this. He said something like, *"Sometimes during sex, it seems like you enjoy me touching your breasts, and sometimes it seems like you hate it."* I told him that's true, because my body has a cycle and a rhythm, and during different parts of my cycle my breasts feel more tender than other times, which is why sometimes I just don't enjoy being touched like that and other times I do. His mind was blown, a light bulb went off, and from that very simple conversation he realised that women's bodies are not the same all the time. My husband is a physiotherapist, a great communicator, and a very curious person – and even with all of the body aware advantages he has, this concept of the fluidity and dynamic nature of a woman's body hadn't landed quite as it seemed to in that moment. I'm certainly not in judgement of him because even as a woman myself, having lived in a woman's body for 36 years, this concept hadn't landed fully for me until I was about 32, and even now I am still learning. What made this interaction an opportunity for powerful communication that helped my partner understand my body and our sex life better was 1) me knowing my body, knowing what I enjoy, and how that can change throughout my cycle, 2) our willingness as individuals to be curious, open and vulnerable and have what can easily feel like an awkward conversation and, 3) my willingness to communicate in my own way what I enjoy and what I don't in the bedroom along with my husband's desire to be aware of that.

To enjoy the pleasure of sex, we need to become curious enough about our bodies and what we enjoy and when. It's not like we take an inventory of what feels good, and use it as a prescription to give to our partners saying, *"Here are all the things that I find enjoyable and pleasurable, and here are all the things that I dislike. Here is a record of my cycle, and when xyz will feel good and this is when it won't. Now go study this and we will have a great sex life."* It doesn't work like that.

If we consider what is required to be able to enjoy the pleasure of sex, we know that being able to communicate what stimulates pleasurable and safe connection is important. Every woman is different in how they feel comfortable expressing what feels good and what doesn't. There isn't one right way to communicate your needs and desires to your partner/s, but there is one essential ingredient and that is vulnerability. We need to lean into that sometimes-uneasy feeling of being vulnerable to be able to communicate in our own way what feels good at any given moment. Being able to communicate our desires also means being willing to stay present in our body during moments of intimacy and sex.

Some questions for clarity:

- How do you communicate with your partner your needs/desires regarding sex?

- Is there a conversation you would like to open more dialogue around?
- What would help you to feel safe to have this vulnerable conversation?

ASKING FOR WHAT YOU WANT AND BEING WILLING TO RECEIVE IT

How willing are you to ask for what you want? Not just in regards to sexual pleasure, but in all aspects of your life? We are all powerful co-creators of our reality, and knowing what you want, being willing to ask for what you want, and being open to receiving it is all part of the creative process.

The first essential step in this creative process is knowing what you want. What do you want from sex and intimacy? Not just on a physical level, but on a spiritual and emotional level too? Consider what it is that you want/need to enjoy sex and intimacy. Some suggestions may be:

- Connection to yourself and your partner
- To feel safe
- Time to feel aroused
- A sense of exploration and adventure
- Body presence
- Vulnerability
- Good communication

How willing are you to ask for what you want? My clients often say that they avoid giving guidance to their partner during sex because they are concerned that they will be misunderstood, that their partner will be insulted thinking that he/she isn't 'good' at pleasuring her, or that they risk being too direct or potentially hurtful. Connecting to the intention behind asking for what you want and why is more powerful than trying to predict another person's reaction.

What is your intention behind asking for what it is you want from sex?

- To open conversation and generate dialogue that helps you grow stronger as an individual and as a couple?
- To create a stronger connection?
- To maximise your experience of pleasure during sex?
- To display to your partner that you feel safe to be vulnerable?
- To practice being vulnerable and honest, expressing yourself, and communicating fully by asking for what you want?
- To explore and find out what it is you want from sex?

When we contemplate our willingness to ask for what we want during sex, and in all aspects of our life, there will be some commonalities of how we tend to act and our underlying beliefs regarding receiving. There may also be some viewpoints that are unique only to sex. These commonalities and the unique views can offer us some valuable insight into what we have accepted as a belief, and may shine some light onto where we have denied our truth and buried it under shame and guilt. Following are some reflections to help bring to the forefront of your awareness where you may be hiding your truth under a veil of shame or guilt.

- How do you feel about asking for what you want during sex?
- How do you feel about asking for what you want in other parts of your life?
- Are there similarities between your willingness to ask for what you want during sex, and in other parts of your life?

- How is asking for what you want during sex different from asking for what you want in other areas in your life?
- Why do you think/feel this is?
- Would you like to be more willing to give direction during sex and intimacy?
- Would you like to be more open to receiving during sex?
- What would asking for what you want during sex look like for you?
- How would asking for what you want during sex this feel for you?
- What would help you feel more willing or able to express your desires during sex?

The reason we said yes to this physical existence is that we knew that in this world we would be able to experience and express a full spectrum of human emotions, and we would be capable of bringing our desires into physical existence. We said yes to our human experience and yes to experiencing pleasure in our body and our being.

We are the creators of our life and our experience. We know about the law of attraction, and we know that when we follow feelings that feel good, we can manifest our desires. The feelings that don't feel good offer us an internal guidance system that essentially shows us when we're following the wrong path and when we focus on those feelings, we also manifest our reality by attracting more of that into our experience.

When we have a desire, we often believe that it is possible and at the same time unlikely. We get in our own way of creation because we turn and look to all of the reasons why that couldn't be possible, we get caught up in 'the how' and we begin to focus on *what isn't rather than what is.* We cut ourselves off from asking for what we want because we begin to believe it's not possible, but at the same time, the desire doesn't go away because it is the desire that is trying to lead us to feel the good feelings that would help us open the door and step closer towards manifesting our desires.

Essentially our desires act as a way of showing us towards feeling good, and feeling good helps us to manifest more of our truth and our desires. When we think about life like this, we can begin to wonder why we don't just ask for what we want. Is it because we are afraid that we won't get it? Is it because we think we don't deserve it? Maybe it's because we are concerned that if we have what we want, we are taking something away from someone else, or we must sacrifice our values or our integrity. All of these concerns are grown in a fear-based reality and one that ultimately stops us from living in alignment with our true nature and our values. We are signing up to what someone else told us to believe is true and possible for us. In short, if we simply had a desire, and were to honour the feelings that would show us our way towards manifesting that desire, we are powerful enough to create the thing but more importantly, we get to feel good in our journey of creation. That is living in alignment with our internal value system. Why then would we shy away from asking for what we want?

BEING OPEN TO RECEIVE

As well as asking for what we want, both during sex and in all aspects of our life, we need to be willing to receive. It's so interesting how our ability to ask for what we want during sex and our willingness to receive pleasure during sex can act as a mirror for our ability or willingness to do the same in all parts of our life.

In the following reflective prompts, you can use the words 'what I want' (or any word/s that resonates) to replace pleasure.

- How willing am I to fully receive pleasure?
- Where in my life am I open to pleasure?
- What does that stimulate and attract for me?
- How do I resist pleasure?

Simple ways to become curious about your willingness to receive and your mindset regarding receiving is to consider behaviours that you may not consciously associate with receiving pleasure. These may be things like:

- How willing are you to ask for and accept help?
- How do you respond to compliments? Do you brush it off? Maybe you say 'Thank you!' but your inner critic tells you that their opinion doesn't count or is offered with poor judgement. Perhaps you say thanks and mean it, but don't actually let the compliment land, you don't let yourself feel the compliment.
- When you hug your partner do you receive the sensation of love and connection, or are you just simply in the habit of giving a hug and kiss goodbye without feeling its full meaning?
- Do you taste your food or just throw it down?

These are all simple times where we get to choose how we receive life and the pleasures that are available to us moment to moment.

If you feel more able to fully receive and open yourself to pleasure in some components of your life, you might find it helpful to consider that receiving energy and contemplate how you can translate that into other aspects of your life. For example, you may take the energy of how you fully connect to your children when you embrace them, and use that energy of connection to allow you to become more present in your body during sex. This has nothing to do with thinking about embracing your children during sex, but it's the energy of that connection that you sense with your children and your willingness to receive their love and embrace that you can invite into other aspects of your life.

We want to enjoy and receive pleasure, connection, and love. We spend much of our time searching for things that will make us feel good. The question is, are you open to receiving what you want? Investing energy in seeking something that you are not open to receive doesn't make sense. How can you open your mind, heart, body, and spirit to receiving what it is you want from sex and life?

SEX AND SENSUALITY IN MOTHERHOOD

Many women, particularly mothers, speak of a desire to increase their libido. Mothers want to desire sex and intimacy with their partners, but sometimes we just don't. Often women notice that this stems from an underlying feeling that their body is undesirable in some way. They describe feeling broken or that disappointed that their body just doesn't look or feel like it used to. An overwhelming sense of vulnerability makes intimacy and sex hard to enjoy.

There is a multitude of things that change when we become parents. Seemingly fleeting moments for possible intimacy and connection, sleep deprivation, redefining who you are as an individual, rediscovering your body after having given birth, creating a new relationship with baby... the list goes on. After birth, women often don't give themselves time to reconnect back to their bodies. I'm not referring to the time that will naturally pass where our body will continue to change and recover after birth. I'm talking about carving out intentional space and time where the intention and focus are on simple body connection. It's a process of rediscovering your body and getting to know and understand your body again. Your body has changed dramatically and in a short period, so it's only natural that we take time to tune in and reconnect with ourselves on all levels; physically, emotionally, sexually, sensually, energetically, and spiritually. Using the practices in this book can be helpful. The essential first step is the acknowledgment and awareness of the need or yearning for this reconnection to take place.

Many women describe a reduced interest in sex after birth, some for months, some for years afterwards. Many mothers attribute this to being tired, hormonal changes, and the fact that we have little people all over us constantly leading to a desire for more space and less touch. This can all be true. However, there is often more to it. Disinterest in sex after birth can develop for a number of reasons including birth trauma, not feeling connected to your body after birth, and stem pelvic floor changes.

When I work with women who experience a disinterest in sex that is related to birth trauma I often witness one of two experiences – pelvic disengagement or overactivation of the pelvic floor. Physically, pelvic disengagement or pelvic dissociation, manifests as reduced pelvic sensation, difficulty activating the muscles of the pelvic floor, challenged pelvic floor co-ordinations, and symptoms of prolapse and incontinence. Women with pelvic disengagement will often describe feeling unable to be present within the pelvic bowl. Alternatively, birth trauma may lead to a protective response within the pelvis, which again manifests physically and energetically but in a different way. Protective activation of the pelvic floor is observed as increased muscle activation and pelvic floor tightness, pelvic pain, and increased sensitivity of the pelvic floor.

A disinterest in sex can also evolve from the body changes that we experience during pregnancy and birth. This may be related to the change in shape or appearance of our body, or related more specifically to pelvic health changes such as incontinence and prolapse.

Many mothers describe feeling that they are no longer whole within their body, they feel broken in some way. When we are unable to connect to our body in a way that feels whole, we become disconnected from our sensual self. When we feel unable to connect to our sensual self, sex feels overwhelming. When we don't feel whole within out body, our connection to joy and pleasure becomes diminished and therefore our connection to sex and the pleasure of sex becomes diminished too.

Even when there is no history of birth trauma, mothers can experience a disinterest in sex that is related to a sense of disconnect from the body. Again, our body has changed dramatically in a short period of time, and when we don't get to know and understand our body after birth it can feel foreign. When we feel foreign in our body, we feel less safe to be vulnerable. We find it very challenging to invite someone into our energetic and physical space because we don't feel safe to do so.

The first step in increasing our interest in sex after birth is recognising that things could feel different and that it is possible to enjoy sex as a mother. Using the body connection practices within this book will help you to be in communication with your body in a way that reveals your path towards improved intimacy and feeling safe in your body sensually and sexually.

7

MOVEMENT AND MOVEMENT MINDSET

Back in the days when we lived much simpler lives, movement was part of our lifestyle, our traditions, and our culture. For many people it still is, but for most of us in the Western world, movement has become structured exercise, often indoors and often led by someone else telling us how to move, for how long, and how many times a week. Of course, this has its value but the concern is that this approach may feed the societal disconnect we have from our emotional, spiritual and physical bodies. Our approach to health, wellbeing, movement, and exercise has become as fast-paced, structured, and disembodied as our lives. We lack exploration and understanding of our body and our mind-body connection.

Working with women in the capacity that I do, more often than not women say they feel disconnected, unsure of their body and often completely broken. Even when women come to me in a state of perceived wellness, when we start to connect inwardly they often discover that they have been living and moving in ways that are more disconnected from their body than they first thought.

If the purpose of movement is to increase our overall wellbeing (spiritual, emotional, and physical), it seems counterintuitive to move our bodies in ways that don't take into consideration things like our hormonal cycle, our creative cycle, our pelvic health, our emotional state, and our energy levels. Women are unique. We are not small men. Our exercise and movement should reflect that.

Don't get me wrong, I believe we can participate in the same sports and leisure activities that men do and that we can excel if we choose to. What I am talking about is the opportunity that is missed when we neglect tuning into our unique rhythm and how many of us find ourselves seeking something more, but never quite knowing what that is. That peaceful sensation of simply feeling at home in our body can seem forever elusive unless we can connect back into our body. One of the most powerful ways in which I know how to do that is through movement. As we engage with more body-led, intuitively guided movement we learn to respect and celebrate our body moving within our own rhythm. When we understand our movement mindset and our mind-body connection, we can carry this insight into other aspects of our life, giving us more clarity around how we can move through our world in a way that reflects more of us.

INTUITIVE MOVEMENT

Intuitive movement is essentially body-led movement. I like to think of body-led movement as a way to explore, express and communicate with your body. It differs from exercise in the sense that the purpose of the movement is to simply *be in* your body rather than working towards a particular goal, like increasing your running pace or dropping some weight.

Moving with the intention of body connection and self-expression is what I believe is at the core of intuitive movement. Intuitive movement is a beautiful way to practice being in touch with your body's rhythm and understand how you like to express yourself in different phases of your cycle.

Body-led movement helps us to create new neural pathways that reinforce patterns of moving through your world by responding to your inner world, rather than moving in certain directions based on perceived expectations. The following practices can help you to invite intuitive movement practices into your life.

MOVEMENT VERSUS EXERCISE

A simple practice is to consider what movement means to you and how it feels. What does exercise mean to you? Perhaps exercise feels more rigid and structured. Movement may feel more free, explorative and fluid. You may like to journal your thoughts. Practice shifting your language from exercise to movement for a couple of weeks and observe what changes for you. Do you move your body differently? Does your relationship with exercise change? What feels different to you?

Connecting to what phrase or term feels good for you helps you to connect with a way to be in your body that feels good to you. We don't need to make exercise wrong and movement right, or vice versa. It's about bringing a simple awareness of how you want to move and feel in your body. From that awareness, you can begin to make choices regarding your physical body movement that feels better to you.

YOUR MOVEMENT INTENTION

What is the intention behind your movement? Understanding the motivation behind your movement can give you insight into your relationship with your body and offer you an opportunity to strengthen that relationship.

What's your movement intention? Are you moving to try and change something about your body? Are you constantly trying to fix something that's not broken? Are you concerned that if you're not exercising in a particular way that your body won't be as appealing? Perhaps you have never considered your intention behind your movement and go through the motions without any particular connection to your body.

Creating an intention for your movement practice can be powerful. You can choose to use a single intention for a period of time, or you can choose to create an intention based on how you feel in the moment. You can create an intention that has a personal focus or a collective focus. For example, an intention with a personal focus may be to feel grounded, and connect to nature during your movement practice. A collective focus may be to express and celebrate your femininity through movement, offering your practice in a way that creates healing energy for women across the globe. There is no right or wrong way to create an intention for your movement practices. Simply tune in and feel for what comes to your heart, mind, or body.

During your movement practices tune back into your chosen intention from time to time. Use it as an anchor to stay present in your practice.

MOVE FOR ENERGETIC NOURISHMENT
- NOT PUNISHMENT

The core belief that you are not good enough as you are and that something needs to change is the motivation behind moving for punishment. The core belief that you deserve to feel good is the motivation behind moving for energetic nourishment.

When we move for energetic nourishment we are moving to feel good, to feel energised, and to feel connected to ourselves and to our body. We are moving for the joy of moving and we are celebrating our body not only for what it can do functionally but for how good it can feel when we express ourselves through movement. When we move for energetic nourishment, it becomes less about how you are performing and the aesthetics of your movement, and more about self-expression.

When we are moving for punishment we are moving because we ate something 'bad', or because we need to lose weight, we are moving because we essentially don't feel good enough. Moving from the energy of punishment reinforces the thought pattern of not being good enough. It keeps us trapped in a cycle that we won't be able to get out of until we establish a new core belief. Alternatively, moving for energetic nourishment reinforces the mindset that we deserve to feel good, so we move. It's the energy behind the movement that allows us to either feel good in our body or continue to feel unworthy and not good enough.

How can you move more for energetic nourishment rather than punishment?

LET THE FEELING FUEL YOUR MOVEMENT

A simple yet powerful way to move from a place of energetic nourishment is to connect with *how you want to feel in your body*. Sit in stillness, breathe into your body and ask yourself, "How do I want to feel?" Once you can connect to how you want to feel, find movement that brings that feeling to life!

HONOUR YOUR BODY AND YOUR NATURAL CYCLES

As human beings, we have a natural rhythm and natural cycles. As women, our cyclical nature can become very obvious when we start to tune into our menstrual cycle. However, our menstrual cycle isn't the *only* cycle that operates within us and around us. We have our creative cycles, seasonal cycles, and our human life cycle just to mention a few. We are constantly transitioning, and our movement practices can reflect our energy at any given phase of any transition or cycle.

I talk more about tuning into your natural rhythm in Part 2: Menstrual Magic. Here I share more specifically about tuning into your natural rhythm and letting that lead your movement. Depending on how you already move your body, and how structured your movement routine is, different pieces of this section will resonate more strongly with you.

As an athlete, I know that, generally speaking, structured training plans don't take into consideration our natural rhythm. Some would argue that training plans do take into consideration the need to rest and recover, and have a cyclical nature to them as structured training plans have foundational phases, building phases, and rest and recovery phases. Essentially though, these phases are created with an outcome in mind, rather than the individual's needs and what phase she is in internally. Even less structured routines that aren't working towards a particular goal can operate at a level where the movement routine is based on an external environment like a gym class timetable, or what day of the week it is, rather than our own internal environment.

When we opt to move in ways that reflect our body's natural rhythm and natural cycles, what we are essentially choosing is to allow ourselves ultimate flexibility in our movement routine. We base our movement practices on how we feel, and how we would like to feel. We choose to base our movement practices on our internal environment, rather than an external system. In the following pages, you will find intuitive movement practices and mindset shifts that will help you connect with your body and help to guide your movement.

DITCH THE TIMETABLE AND MEASUREMENTS

There is nothing wrong with structure and routine. Some people thrive within these conditions. However, when you are exploring intuitive and body-led movement practices, particularly in the early phases, taking away the timetable is useful.

When we stick to schedules, we are essentially asking ourselves to comply with an external motivator that directs our movement practices. Monday is boxing, Tuesday is Pump class, Wednesday is yoga, Thursday a run...Tuning into your body and practicing body-led movement requires us to move from within by using our internal compass to direct our movement.

We become more able to let our body guide us in how we can move for energetic nourishment. Tuning in to your own body's rhythm means asking your body simple questions like, "How would you like to move today?" as opposed to thinking, "Today is Tuesday, so I run."

Even if you're sticking to the same kind of movement practice each day – take running for example - you can ask your body to take the lead on guiding the distance, the time, the pace, and the intensity.

In group settings, many women feel the pressure to keep up with other class participants. Ditching the measurements also means ditching the comparison to others. If you truly want to explore intuitive and body-led movement trying to keep up with someone else's performance will not serve you. Using your body to guide your movement is what this is all about.

Lose the watches, the timers, the scales, and any other external measure that shifts your focus from body presence to external expectations. These measurements hold little value in helping you to tune inwardly. When we focus on pace, distance, or time we are holding ourselves to expectations, rather than letting our body guide us. You don't need to let them go forever. It can be a conscious choice you make for a period of time to see how your body responds and how you feel.

INVITE VARIETY

Often, we find ourselves moving in the same ways over and over again. This can happen for various reasons. Perhaps we prefer a particular kind of movement practice and we have become stuck in our ways. It can be because we believe there is one 'correct' way of doing a particular task and so we strive for doing it correctly, rather than simply experimenting with our movement. It could be that we have never challenged ourselves to be more creative with how we move. There is nothing wrong with consistent movement patterns, but in doing this we may be giving ourselves less opportunity to build our body's resilience. When we invite variety into our movement practice, we create more opportunities for our body to move differently, which helps to grow resilience. Movement variability also helps to grow our mind and body's flexibility.

Inviting variety into your movement doesn't require you to sign up to *all* of the things. It can be as simple as experimenting with different ways of moving your body in the comfort of your home, in your natural environment, or even in group classes that you may already be attending. There are so many ways you can create more variety in your movement. Here are some examples:

- Slow your pace, particularly if you're accustomed to moving in hard and fast ways. If you love to get sweaty, it can be challenging to slow down your movement but slowing down can create a sense of connectedness with your body that fast movement might not. Slow movement often invites more body awareness and presence.

- Decrease your range of movement. Again, if you're used to big movements it can be challenging to move within a smaller range. We often think bigger is better. When you allow yourself to move within a smaller range you may find that smaller movements can actually be more challenging.

- Change your direction. Take walking for example; walk backwards, or sideways instead of forward all the time. Try this up and down stairs. Instead of always doing forward lunges, take them backward and sideways as well. You can bring more angles into your movement with simple experimentation.

- If you lift weights, rather than always using evenly weighted equipment, try some movements with uneven weights. This is an excellent challenge.

- Rather than using store-bought equipment, take yourself out of the gym and begin to practice out in nature instead. Use your imagination. Experiment with rocks, trees, trails, and natural inclines.

- Get onto the web and look up different movement practices to try. It's free and easily accessible. Try a Barre class, yoga, Pilates, boxing, or some running drills. Open your mind, have fun, and simply experiment.

- Challenge yourself to find ways that you can change your practiced movement patterns. Take a simple squat for example. How can you practice this movement in different ways? There's more than one way to squat, though many of us have been taught there is only one 'right' way. Moving in only one particular pattern doesn't reflect how we are required to move our body in the real world. Challenge your movement patterns by changing your posture and technique.

Inviting movement variety is as simple as taking yourself out of your practiced zone. Challenge yourself with something a little different.

CONNECT BACK TO YOUR CHILDHOOD PASSION

I find it so fascinating how many women say to me, "I used to love dancing. It was my thing. I guess I just stopped one day and never started again. You know, when I think about what kind of movement would light me up and feel good in my body it's dancing. Which makes me wonder why I'm going to the gym?"

Of course, it's not always dancing, but the essence is the same. Somewhere along the line we lost connection to what movement feels good to us, and have instead subscribed to a program that someone else told us would be good for us. Often, the underlying reason why we despise exercise or find it hard to motivate ourselves to move our body is that we aren't allowing ourselves to choose movement that feels good.

Connect back to your childhood passion. One caution: when you do this, remember not to approach this with expectation and comparison to what you were once able to do. Your body will be different, and your ability to perform particular skills might have changed. Approach with fun and lightness rather than judgement and criticism.

MOVE TO YOUR RHYTHM

One of the simplest ways to help you tune into your body's rhythm is to tune into the music. What kind of music do you feel like listening to right now? Something chilled and laid back? Or do you prefer something upbeat with some rhythm right now? Simply asking yourself what type of music you would like to listen to, and moving your body in a way that reflects the rhythm and flow of the music helps to access our body's intuition with ease.

SUPER SIMPLE BODY LED MOVEMENT

- Take a four-point kneeling position.
- Close the eyes and connect to the breath.
- Bring your awareness to your body, finding areas of spaciousness and perhaps areas of tension.
- Ask your body how it would like to move.
- Begin to move your body in ways that feel expressive and nourishing.
- Practice being in your body, without your movement having to evolve to anything in particular.
- Let your body lead your movement without having to fulfill a goal, without trying to change something about your body, and without trying to perfect or correct how you move.

You don't need to stay in the four-point kneeling position. It's simply a suggestion of a nice place to start. Other nice starting positions are standing, lying with the knees bent and feet flat on the floor, and sitting with the legs crossed.

RADICAL REST IS REQUIRED

Practicing slowness and stillness can be particularly challenging for women who are natural or well-practiced movers. Women who are self-motivated and move through their life with ambition and drive can find it difficult to slow down. Slowing down can feel scary for some of us! This may be because we equate our value to our productivity, which is something to become curious about in itself.

It may also be that we are subconsciously or even consciously concerned about what might happen if we actually slow down. The fear of slowing down can be palpable for women who are in some way addicted to being constantly 'on'. Some worry that if they slow down, they would realise how good that actually feels and that maybe they would never start again. Others are concerned about losing control because slowing down might mean others may need to help, and accepting help from others means that things won't get done in the exact same way we would do it.

Slowing down and offering opportunities for stillness in small doses is a nice way to begin. Once we can feel the benefits, we naturally invite more stillness, slowness, and simplicity into our lives. We don't need to wrong our motivation and our ability to take action. That's a gift to be admired and appreciated. It's about taking time to reflect on how we feel and being honest with ourselves. If we keep expecting ourselves to keep on keeping on when we are tired or edging on burn out, we are unable to nourish our being in a way that we are then able to be of best service to ourselves and others.

When it comes to movement, the dominating messages are those of consistency and persistence and the need to keep active. This is true - we do need to keep active for our wellbeing - but that doesn't reduce the value of rest. Rest is phenomenally valuable, particularly for those of us who are self-motivated seekers. Practicing radical rest in how we physically move our body is a nice way to sense the slowness and our resistance to it.

My work as a physiotherapist and my experience as a high-level athlete provides endless examples of how we fail to thrive when we don't allow ourselves to rest. The injury that never quite resolves because it wasn't given the time to heal; the numerous athletes interviewed at the end of their career being asked, "What's the one thing you wish you had learned earlier in your career?" who respond with "To listen to my body and learn to rest". I'm sure if I asked you to remember an experience where you neglected the value of rest and ignored your body's messages, it wouldn't take you long to think of one. We can generally follow up with some reason why we couldn't rest – there was a deadline, there was an important competition coming up, you were getting bored and frustrated. For many of us, learning the value of rest requires us to experiment with it long enough to experience the effects. It requires us to be willing to experience the uncomfortable feelings that resting brings up in us for long enough to see the positive side effects. Until we experience the effects of rest, we are so resistant to it that we are unable to open our minds to a new way and a new possibility that rest can be helpful, rather than a hindrance.

The challenge many of us face is not to keep moving, but to *rest, reset, and recalibrate*. These states are all part of our natural rhythm, and once we embrace rest we will start to see how much we need it, and how much better off we are for taking it.

INCORPORATING REST

What is your relationship with rest? What are your beliefs around rest? Contemplate and write them down or talk it out with a friend.

In relationship to movement:

- How willing are you to take a 'rest day' from your training?
- Do you rest when you feel tired, worn-out, or injured?
- What does rest look like and feel like to you?
- What language do you use around resting? Is it positive or negative? Do you recognise these phrases? No pain - no gain, no excuses, cheat day, lazy OR restorative, necessary, deserved?

- Are you always in active recovery? Only allowing rest for the purpose of recovery? Only resting after the work is done?

In relationship to your entire life:

- How do I honour my need for rest?
- What does rest look like and feel like for me?
- If I could embrace rest more, without a sense of guilt, how would that feel? How would that look?
- When I feel rested, life looks like..? Life feels like...?
- When I don't feel well rested, life looks like...? Life feels like...?
- What would have me feel safe and supported to embrace my need for rest more?

Let yourself tune in to your body and notice how it is feeling, allow yourself to experiment with responding in a way that feels nourishing. Take a simple first step towards experimenting with rest.
This could look like:

- Sitting still for just a couple of minutes without finding something to distract you
- Slowing the pace of your movement
- Stopping and taking five slow, deep breaths
- Saying no to something
- Choosing a nap, even when that feels uncomfortable
- Following your active recovery plan, without ramping up the intensity

MOVEMENT & MOVEMENT MINDSET
JOURNAL PROMPTS

- How would I like movement to feel?
- How would movement for energetic nourishment look/feel like?
- How do my movement practices reflect my body's natural rhythm and cycles
- If I honoured my body's natural rhythm and cycles, what would movement look/feel like?
- What ignites movement momentum and movement motivation within?
- What movement practices would I like to explore, but haven't yet?
- What holds me back from exploring different ways of moving my body?
- If I was to let go of these stories, and allow myself to explore movement as a way of connecting with my body, what would I be doing?
- How can I feel safe and supported in my movement practices?
- How do I feel about resting my body?
- What do I sense are the benefits of rest?
- When I contemplate body-led/intuitive movement, what fears arise for me? What do I sense this means about my relations with my body?
- If I could trust that my body knows the way, what action/in-action would I be taking?
- If I embraced a more intuitive style of movement what would that look/feel like for me?
- What feels important to me when it comes to movement? How can I honour that?

8

BODY CONNECTION
PRACTICES

SETTING A SACRED SPACE

Having a sacred space for your self-connection practices and rituals can help to maintain the momentum of your practice by giving you a physical anchor point, a gentle reminder to encourage the habit of practice, and a retreat for you to enjoy. By using your space with some consistency, you begin to create ritual for yourself, which can add to the meaning and feeling of sacredness to your practice. Your sacred space doesn't need to be particularly big nor fancy. My most precious sacred spaces have existed in a small backyard, in my bedroom, and my patient/client clinic room.

When choosing a space in your home that feels right for you, you may like to consider how you feel in that space, the amount of privacy it offers, and if you will be able to access the space during the times that will suit you to practice. Of course, there is no right or wrong way to set up your space. Here I will give you a few suggestions of how you can make your space feel unique and special to you without too much effort or expense. After all, it's the practice that matters most and the power comes from within you, not any crystals or cards that you may choose to use as an adjunct to the practice.

First, consider how you would like to feel in your space. What would you like to see, feel, taste, and hear? Are there any precious things that you feel connected to that would help to make your space feel sacred? What would make this space feel safe, comfortable, and inviting for you?

Some things that I use are:

- Yoga mat
- Pillows/bolster
- Blanket

- Eye pillow (or rice bag wrapped in a scarf)
- Candles
- Oils and a diffuser
- Oracle/tarot cards/daily inspiration cards
- Crystals
- Journal
- Inspirational book/s (check out your local library)

Your sacred space doesn't need to have anything special in it. It just needs to feel good for you. When I can, I like to do my practices outside. Here I can feel the elements and enjoy connecting with nature. My back yard becomes my sacred space, which is super simple – just me and nature.

CREATING THE TIME

One of the biggest perceived barriers to practicing self-connection, movement, and self-care is time, particularly for mothers. Often, it's because we sense a need or a desire for solitude to be able to embody a particular depth in our practice, but this is not always a possibility. This can create a push/pull sensation within and lead to frustration and guilt. Sometimes the yearning for solitude takes us away from our practice or our sense of being able to be present during our practice. We become so focused on trying to manipulate our surroundings and our environment that we take ourselves out of being present by simply being in the practice no matter what that looks like. On top of that, the yearning for solitude can take us out of being present as a mother because we are fixated on looking for an escape. If we take time to challenge our perspective here, we can find that the opportunity exists for us to find even more depth to our practice while being present as a mother by simply asking ourselves what is the purpose of the practice? The purpose is to be present with our body, our self, and with whatever is here for us in this moment. Of course, solitude gifts us the space to calm the mind, connect to the breath and drop into our body but we practice this in solitude/silence so that we can invite these embodied ways of being into our day-to-day life. The gift of motherhood can mean that we practice with the fluidity and flexibility that life requires, rather than trying to control our life and circumstances. As mothers, particularly with small children, the moments we have on our own can be rare, but it's often our unwillingness to practice in circumstances that we don't see as perfect or desirable that limits our potential. We spend too much time trying to manipulate our circumstances, rather than simply immersing ourselves in the practice when it feels good. This isn't something to beat ourselves up about, rather it is something to simply acknowledge and challenge.

Small moments of practice can create powerful effects. We sometimes forget that we don't need an hour, but maybe just a few minutes. We can get caught up in all of the reasons why we can't: "It will only be five minutes before the kids come in and distract me again". Take five minutes! Don't forget the law of attraction. When we gift ourselves these moments in time, we tend to be gifted more of these moments in unexpected ways. Say yes to your practice by accepting how it looks at any given moment, and notice the power of imperfect practice.

IGNITE YOUR SENSES

Igniting our senses can be a powerful way of creating neural pathways, just like the experiment with Pavlov's Dog. In the famous experiment, Pavlov found that objects or events could trigger a conditioned response. Pavlov designed an experiment using a bell as a neural stimulus. As he gave food to the dogs, he rang the bell. Then, after repeating this procedure, he tried ringing the bell without providing food to the dogs. On its own, the dog began to salivate. The result of the experiment was a new conditioned response in the dogs.

How you choose to ignite your senses is going to be very personal. You may want to focus on visual stimuli if you know you're a visual person, or touch if you know you're more tactile. The trick is to add these stimuli to your personal practices, and then integrate their use in your day-to-day life. Repetition of sensory input builds sensory pathways. By integrating sensory input into your personal practices, you begin to ingrain a hugely positive association with these inputs. Outside of your dedicated practice, these sensory tools can act as an anchor point to help you bring you back to the present moment in your day to day life.

Let me give you some ideas on how you can do this. Once you've felt into what resonates with you, you can start to implement its use in your practices and into your day-to-day living.

SOUND

Does music fill your soul? Add music to your movement, meditation, and mindfulness practice, using the same piece of music for a period of time. Playing your chosen music in your day-to-day can then act as reminder to slow down, connect with the body and notice how you feel. Of course, this is just one example of how you can use this practice - be creative and use your intuition.

SCENT

Scents can create very positive associations for us. Imagine the smell of Christmas, or your favourite holiday destination. Scent can be very powerful - and we can easily integrate it into our practice.

Essential oils and candles are just two examples of how you can do this. Integrating the use of oils in your meditation, massage, or movement practices, and then using them throughout your day can help to act as an anchor point to come back to.

Integrate oils to your tuning in practice and, as you breathe deeply, enjoy the scent. Then continue to use this oil during the day as a gentle reminder to tune in and be present. I like to use candles during my slower movement practices, as well as during my self-massage and journaling. During the day I burn a few candles around the house and when I see them it acts as a great reminder to slow down, breathe, and tune in.

TOUCH

Touching your heart or your womb space can anchor you back into your body. Using touch throughout the day is a super simple way to stay grounded and connected. Noticing your sensations is another. Feel the breeze on your face, feel the sweat running down your legs, and feel the sand on the beach as you walk barefoot.

Combine any of the above techniques. Experiment with them all, and see what works for you. Be creative and keep an open mind. If your instinct or intuition tells you to try something, go with it. These impulses come to us for a reason!

BODY SCAN PRACTICE

This simple practice is designed to help you tune into your body's energy. You can use this to help guide your movement practices, your day to day tasks, and to invite more body-led living into your life. This is also a nice practice to bring awareness to your body and to note any areas that you may be holding tension- this is particularly helpful if you experience pelvic pain due to overactive muscles of the deep core. As you scan your body and notice areas of tension, invite your body to relax and release. You can do this during simple day to day tasks like washing up, sitting at your computer, or lying in bed at night. By regularly checking in with your physical body, you can become more aware of when you may be holding your body with more effort than is required.

- Bring yourself to a comfortable and relaxed position. Lying flat on your back or sitting in a chair with your feet supported are desirable positions when starting with this practice. Over time, as you become more familiar with the practice, you can perform a body scan in moments wherever you are.
- Gently close the eyes and bring your awareness to your breath.
- Breathing in and out through your nose, begin to notice the noises outside the room/space you are in. Then bring your awareness to the space you are in, noticing the sounds that surround you.
- Notice the temperature of the room, the temperature of your body, the clothes on your skin, where you feel them touching you, your breath and how the body expands and fills with each breath in, how the body softens and relaxes with each breath out. Notice your entire body.
- Then begin to scan the body, starting with the crown of your head, tuning into the sensations within the body. Notice where your body feels spacious and relaxed, and where you feel as though it is holding tension.
- Continue to scan your body slowly, moving your awareness downwards to the face, neck, shoulders, chest, arms, elbows, wrists, hands, fingers, abdomen, pelvis, hips, spine, buttocks, thighs, knees, lower legs, ankles, feet and toes. If you find an area of tension, invite this space to soften by gently guiding

your breath towards that space in your body. Notice if you begin to feel self-judgement, and when you might begin to create a dialogue to explain how you feel. Bring the awareness back to the breath and to the body.

- Then notice the entire body as a whole, and how you feel overall.
- You may like to ask your body a simple question like: What do I need? Or what would help me feel supported and nourished? Allow your body to show you how to best support yourself in this moment. Allow the answer to come naturally. Don't force it in any direction. Permit yourself to let your body lead, even when its direction feels unusual or as if it won't be productive or effective. Trust your body, and see how that feels for you.

DEEP CORE CONNECTION PRACTICE (DCCP)

This practice is designed to help you tune into the muscles of the deep core, and begin to notice how your body moves with the breath. This is a simple body awareness practice that creates a beautiful foundation from which your core connection practices can grow.

PART ONE

1) Take your preferred lying position:

- Flat on your back with the legs slightly wider than hip-distance, letting the feet fall softly outwards
- On your back with the knees bent and feet resting flat on your mat. Take the feet wide and let the knees fall into one another.

- Bring the soles of the feet to touch and let the knees fall wide into a butterfly position. Use pillows, rolled blankets/towel, blocks, or bolsters to support the knees if desired

If it feels comfortable, you can make the following hand gesture.

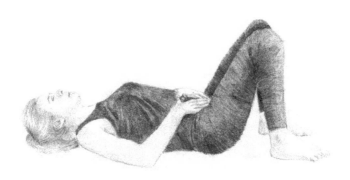

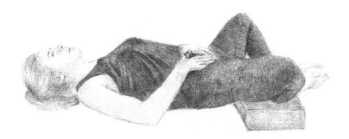

- Bring the thumbs to touch and press the tips of the index fingers together to create a triangle with the hands. Bring the tips of your fingers to rest onto your pubic bone, and the heels of the hands to rest towards the hips.

2) Close the eyes and bring your awareness to your breath, breathing in and out through the nose.

- Begin to trace the breath as it enters the nose and travels down the back of the throat and into the lungs, sensing the movement of the rib cage.

- Particularly notice the front, side, and back of your rib cage as it expands with each inhale and then gently recoils and relaxes with each exhale.
- Stay here for a few minutes, simply being in tune with the breathe and the sensation of the movement of the rib cage with each breath.

3) Bring your awareness to the belly.

- Begin by sensing the movement of the belly with the breath.
- Allow the belly to bulge with each inhale and feel the abdomen gently deflate, feeling the belly button drawing towards the spine with each exhale.
- There is no need to force a contraction. Simply allow yourself to notice how your body moves with the breath with no particular effort.
- If you find it difficult to bring the breath into the belly, you may like to try a gentle springing technique. Take one hand to rest over the abdomen and with each breath out place a gentle pressure onto the abdomen by pressing the hand softly into the belly. As you draw the breath in, focus on breathing into your hand. As you breath into your hand, allow the pressure to gently build and then to be released - feeling a springing sensation at the abdomen. Once you have done this a couple of times, place the hands back into the inverted triangle position (or chosen rest position) and continue to focus on belly breathing for a couple more breaths.

4) Bring your awareness now to your pelvic floor.

- Sense the diamond shape that is created by the muscles of the pelvic floor by imagining the pubic bone at the front of the pelvis, the coccyx at the back and the sit bones on either side.
- Breathe deep into the pelvic bowl, focusing your breath all the way into the perineal space that sits between the vagina and the anus.
- As you breathe in, feel the muscles of the pelvic floor soften and relax. Sense how the pelvic floor muscles open and allow space for the breath. As you breathe out, sense the gentle movement of the pelvic floor as the muscles draw inwards and upwards.
- Again, no particular effort is required to contract the muscles, simply notice how the body moves with the breath.

This is a beautiful stand-alone practice, particularly as you begin to tune into this space. As you become more practiced, your ability to tune into the movement of your body with the breath will become easier. This practice can then become a simple starting point for other extended practices described in this book.

PART TWO

To complete this practice, reverse the practice in the same way as you softened into the pelvic space. Simply draw your awareness back to the belly for a couple more belly breaths; then back to the rib cage, noticing the expansion and softening of the rib cage; then back to the throat, noticing the movement of the breath as it massages the throat space. When you are ready, introduce some gentle movement back into the body in any way that feels good.

PELVIC BOWL AWARENESS PRACTICE

This practice is designed to help you tune into your pelvic bowl energy. Begin this practice with Part One of the Deep Core Connection Practice.

- Once you have tuned into your pelvic floor and the movement of the pelvic floor with the breath, begin to 'clock around' the pelvic bowl with your mind's eye.
- Begin at the pubic bone at the front of the pelvis. Notice the quality of the energy here. Notice where you sense the energy of this space begins and where it seems to end. Notice any sensations that arise in this space.
- Then bring your awareness to the right hipbone at the front of your pelvis, again noticing the quality of the energy here, where it begins and where it ends, along with any sensations that arise.
- Continue with this same simple awareness as you clock around your pelvic bowl; from the right hip bone to the right side of your sacrum at the back, to the right sit bone, to the coccyx in the centre, to the left side of your sacrum, to your left sit bone, to your left hip bone at the front of your pelvis, and back to your pubic bone.
- Then bring your awareness to the entire pelvic bowl while inviting your breath to fill to the edges of your pelvis.

Take time to simply notice the energy of your pelvic bowl and any sensations that may arise during this practice. As you embody this practice, you may like to:

- Ask your body "How can I best nourish myself today?"

- Connect to a simple intention that may arise during this practice
- Begin to explore how your core energy responds to a particular question you may have by sensing if your muscles contract or expand.
- Simply allow whatever comes up to be there, and gently explore in a way that feels safe for you.

Remember there is no right or wrong way to use these practices. Trust whatever feels right for you.

TUNING INTO YOUR OVARY AND WOMB ENERGY

You can use this practice as an extension of the DCCP, or the Pelvic Bowl Awareness Practice. This practice will help you to notice how balanced you are in your life in regards to your 'doing' and 'being' energy. This doesn't mean that you always need to be equal parts of doing and being. The energy within the ovaries and womb space can simply act as a guide to help you know how you may best nourish your being and when your life may have tilted significantly out of balance.

- Once you have tuned into your core energy using the DCCP, bring your awareness to your left ovary and the space in your body that you sense is occupied by your left ovary (even if you have had an ovary or your uterus removed, the energy of these organs will remain).
- Our left ovary energy represents our 'being' energy, our feminine energy; our willingness to nurture ourselves, live in accordance to our body's rhythm, to honour our body's cycles, to rest, and to restore.

- Sense the quality of the energy here. Where does it begin? Where does it end? You may feel a buzzing sensation, a warmth, a coolness, you may feel emptiness, or you may sense nothing at all. There is no right or wrong thing to feel.
- As you sense into the energy of this space, reflect on what this may signify and mean for you. Remember that there is nothing that you need to do to fix or change what you sense, simply notice how you are feeling and what you are sensing.
- Then, bring your awareness to your right ovary energy. This represents our more masculine energy and our willingness to take action, create and honour loving boundaries, and to act in ways that are aligned with our truth. The right ovary can reflect our 'doing' energy. Again, sense into the quality of the energy of this space. Notice where it begins and where it ends, taking some time to reflect on what the sensations that are present mean or represent to you.
- Now bring your awareness to your womb space, feeling into your deep energy centre between the ovaries. Notice how this space in your body feels. Notice the quality of the energy of this space. Taking some time to contemplate and reflect on whatever may be present in this space for you in this moment. Approach with a simple and gentle curiosity.
- This is an opportunity to simply connect with the energy of your centre, noticing how it feels to be in connection and communication with your body. Trust whatever comes up and is present for you.
- As you stay with this space in your body, allow yourself to simply sense whatever may be here for you. Perhaps an intention comes to mind. Perhaps something that you would like to release or let go of becomes apparent. Maybe a new way of being that you would like to begin to embody is sparked. There

is no right or wrong thing to feel. Simply be with whatever is. *That is the practice.*

WOMB MASSAGE

This Womb Massage Practice is designed to help you to create both a physical and energetic connection to your pelvic bowl and womb space. Women often avoid touching themselves in this region of their body, sometimes because they feel some form of shame around this part of their body. Giving simple loving and kind attention to this space creates the potential for a new kind of connection. Go at your own pace and, again, remember there is no way that you can get this wrong. If it feels good and nourishing to you, then you are doing it right. If you do have a newly formed scar or incision site, in the case of a C-section scar for example, be sure that the incision has adequately healed for scar massage to be performed. Generally speaking, massage is beneficial for healthy scar formation and healing once the incision site has adequately healed.

Here are some simple tips to consider when practicing Womb Massage:

SET UP
Suggested positions include:

- On your back with pillows supporting the head and underneath the knees
- On your back with the knees bent and feet rested flat on your mat. Take the feet as wide as your mat and let the knees fall into one another.

- Bring the soles of the feet to touch and let the knees fall wide into a butterfly position and using pillows or rolled blankets/ towel blocks or bolsters to support the knees if desired.

OILS / LOTIONS

For your Womb Massage I recommend that you use some kind of oil, simply because it feels nourishing, though certainly a lotion or cream will work effectively too. Personally, I like to create my own 'Womb Oil' blend using warming oils (such as Cassia) and calming oils (such as Bergamot, Ylang Ylang and Lavender) in a fractionated coconut oil base. Clary Sage is a beautiful oil that is commonly found in Womb Oil blends due to its capacity to relax the uterus. **Be mindful though that it is not recommended to be used during pregnancy or if you are hoping to become pregnant.** Grounding oils such as Frankincense or Sandalwood complement the intention of Womb Massage beautifully too.

ROOM SET UP

A quiet and private space is desirable for womb massage. Here I will offer some suggestions of how to create a calming space for your self-massage (or any of the practices in this book) but you don't actually need any equipment/particular set up to begin this practice. Sometimes not having an ideal space creates a barrier to engaging with these practices, but a commitment to simply explore the practice with the resources you have available is the only thing you need.

- Consider the room temperature - you don't want to feel cold during this practice so blankets or a heater may be required to help you stay comfortable.
- Wearing no underwear is ideal, as you want to be able to access at least to your pubic bone comfortably.

- Low lighting is preferred.

Other beautiful adjuncts to create a soothing and sacred space include:

- Candles
- Soft and calming music
- A journal for afterward to record any musings/thoughts that come to mind during your massage

You can use any pressure that feels comfortable to you. Some massage techniques that you may like to explore are:

- Cross patterning strokes beginning at your rib cage and coming across the body to the opposite hip. For example, using your left hand begin at the right rib cage and stroke the hand towards the left hip bone and vice versa.
- Using the palm to stroke from one side of the abdomen to the other – starting at the bra line working your way down slowly to the pubic bone
- Using the palm of the hands, starting on the perimeter of the torso and stroking towards the navel while imagining a circle and bringing the hand/s from the perimeter of the circle to the navel with each stroke. You may like to imagine that you are bringing any 'leaked energy' that has escaped you back to your centre.
- Creating small circles with the tips of the index and middle finger over the ovaries.
- Starting with the hands resting together between your navel and pubic bone, gently sweep the hands across your pelvis and/or abdomen and towards the ground beneath you. You

may like to imagine 'letting go' of anything that no longer serves you as you do this.

Simply experiment and see what feels good for you.

HEART WOMB CONNECTION

Spending a lot of time focusing on womb space is a powerful practice. Women often describe a sensation of coming home to their body and feeling sensations of peaceful presence that they didn't know was so easily accessible to them. Sometimes though, we can focus so much attention on our womb space without feeling its connection to other powerful spaces in our body like our heart. This very simple practice helps us to bring the heart and womb energy into communication with one another, helping us to further sense the peaceful and pleasant sensations that come from these practices, as well as igniting a deeper level of connectedness to our self and our wholeness.

- Find your comfortable position either sitting, standing, or laying in one of the womb meditation positions described earlier in the DCCP.
- Place one hand onto womb space, and one onto heart space. Gently close the eyes and begin to focus on your breath.
- Breathe into your heart space, feeling the energy of your heart space and being with the sensations that are present for you for a few moments. Let these sensations wash over you.
- Begin to breathe deep down to the pelvic bowl. Focus now on the energy of the pelvic bowl, and being with the sensations that are present for you in this part of your body. Let these sensations wash over your body for a few moments.

- Bring your awareness from your womb space to meet the energy of your heart space. Follow this by bringing the energy of your heart to meet the energy of your womb. Spend some time shifting the focus from womb energy, to the heart, and back to womb. Then sense their energy as a whole within your centre.
- Finally, bring your awareness back to the breath, breathing into the heart and womb space at the same time. If you feel called to, you may like to ask your body what it may need to feel nourished, replenished, and supported. Or you may wish to ask your body for guidance.
- To finish, gently acknowledge yourself for showing up to this practice, and thanking your body.

GETTING FAMILIAR WITH YOUR FEMININE BODY

Getting to know your body, whether after birth or any of the many transition phases that we go through as women, takes willingness and courage. One of the reasons why women avoid getting to know their body intimately is that they are afraid of what they will discover. We are afraid to look at our body because we are worried that we will see won't be 'normal', even though we know that every woman's body is different, and what we are exposed to as a society is an unrealistic depiction of what a woman's body looks like, or is supposed to look like.

We are afraid to experiment with ourselves sexually because we feel dirty or shameful. Sometimes we avoid self-pleasure because we are afraid that things won't 'work' like they used to. Some women have seldom even 'gone there' because they feel shame in self-pleasure. That itself is something to become curious about.

It's often the fear of the unknown that holds us hostage in our body. Once we allow ourselves to explore with simple curiosity we can begin the journey of getting to know our body more intimately, both sexually and non-sexually. If you can take away the fear and the expectation of things to look or be a certain way, and instead take an approach of gentle curiosity, you can begin to find freedom in your body.

One way to become more intimately aware of your body is by simply understanding your female anatomy. Taking a mirror and looking at your vulva and beginning to understand what you see is an excellent first step and this practice will help you do that.

- Sitting (option to sit supported against a wall with a pillow/s to support your back), bend your knees take your feet and knees wide, and use a mirror to begin to explore your feminine body.
- Notice the perineal body - the skin that sits between the anus and the vagina. If you have had a vaginal birth and an episiotomy/tearing, you may notice some scar tissue here. You can breathe deeply into this space and observe any movement here.
- Notice the labia majora – the outer labia.
- Notice the labia minora – the inner labia. Although named the labia minora, they are not necessarily smaller than the labia majora.
- Then, separate the labia and take a look at the entrance to the vagina, the urethra, and the clitoris.
- In this position, you may like to try some pelvic floor contractions and see if you can notice the drawing inward and upward of the perineum and the tightening of the muscles around the entrance of the vagina.

- Notice your urethra, where urine is expelled.
- Notice the clitoral hood and the clitoris itself.

This practice is simply about becoming familiar with the different parts of your feminine body. As you explore this space, you may like to reflect on the pleasure that this space brings you, the beauty of this space, and the power of your feminine body.

VULVA

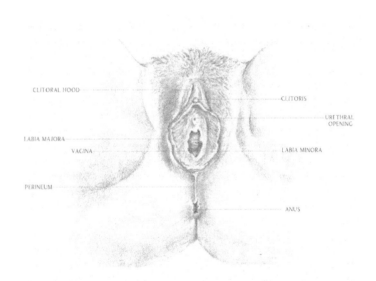

CLITORAL HOOD

CLITORIS

URETHRAL OPENING

LABIA MAJORA

VAGINA

LABIA MINORA

PERINEUM

ANUS

PELVIC FLOOR SELF-MASSAGE

Internal pelvic massage is a simple way that you can become more attuned to and aware of your pelvic health. Internal pelvic massage is a beautiful way to help the muscles of the pelvic floor to relax, as well as for you to have an opportunity to sense the energy within your pelvic bowl on a physical and emotional level.

As long as you are gentle with your body, don't push through any pain, and of course, use good hygiene practices, there is no real right or wrong way to do pelvic self- massage. There are some particular landmarks within the pelvic bowl that practitioners need to avoid due to potential pain and nerve irritation, but when conducting this kind of massage on yourself it's best to simply let your body guide you.

- Generally, the most comfortable position for self-massage is to be reclined with the knees bent and falling wide. Nice places to experiment with pelvic self-massage are in the bathtub if you have one, or reclined in bed with pillows to support you.
- You can choose to use a single finger or thumb for your massage.
- Gently insert your thumb/finger into the vagina, and simply breathe into the pelvic bowl. See if you can sense the movement of your pelvic floor with your breath, feeling a gentle lift as you breathe out, and a relaxing of the muscles with each breath in.
- To explore the left- and right-hand sides of the internal pelvic bowl, it is generally most comfortable if you use the opposite hand to the side of the pelvic bowl that you are exploring. For example, if you are exploring the left side of the pelvic bowl, you would use your right hand.

- To explore the left- and right-hand sides of the pelvic bowl, shift your thumb/finger toward one side of the pelvis. As you do this, avoid pressing onto your urethra because this can be uncomfortable. Place a gentle pressure onto the muscles of the pelvic floor and use a sweeping motion to move your thumb/finger from the front of your pelvis towards the back of your pelvis.
- If you find an area that feels particularly tender, or like it is holding tension, you may like to stop and simply breathe into the space where you can feel the pressure within the pelvis.
- Then, take the opposite hand and gently insert the thumb or finger into the vagina, repeating the pelvic massage on the opposite side of the pelvic bowl. Again, use the sweeping motions, and stop at any particular points of tension and simply breathe into the space in your body where you feel your thumb's gentle pressure.
- As you massage the right side of your pelvic bowl you may wish to contemplate your masculine 'doing' energy, and how you are showing up and sharing with the world. As you massage the left side of your pelvis you may wish to contemplate what it is that you are currently creating, and aspects of your feminine 'being' energy.
- You may like to ask your body how it would best be nourished at this time. Simply wait for the answer.
- Once you have removed your thumb and completed your Pelvic Bowl Self Massage, take a few deep nourishing breaths into the pelvic bowl and simply notice any changes in physical sensations and how you feel emotionally and energetically.

PELVIC FLOOR MASSAGE

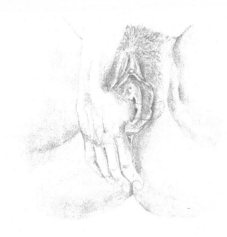

ALTERNATE NOSTRIL BREATHING AND
PELVIC BOWL BALANCING

This is a beautiful practice to use when you feel out of balance, overwhelmed, or stressed. It's also a great practice to use when you have been sitting in your masculine 'doing' energy for a while and would like to invite some calm and ease-filled feminine energy into your mind and body. It will also work in an alternate way if you have been sitting in your 'being' energy for a while and would like to invite some action-taking masculine energy into your life.

Take your preferred position:

- Flat on your back with the legs slightly wider than hip-distance apart, letting the feet fall softly outwards.
- On your back with the knees bent and feet resting flat on your mat. Take the feet as wide as your mat and let the knees fall into one another
- Bring the soles of the feet to touch and let the knees fall wide, using pillows or rolled blankets/towel blocks or bolsters to support the knees if desired.
- When you are comfortable, close the eyes if it feels good and bring your focus to your breath as you breathe in and out through the nose. Let your body relax and the belly bulge with the breath.
- Next take your right hand and create a pistol grip. Bring your hand to your face and press your thumb to your right nostril, so that you begin to breathe through your left nostril only. As you breathe into your left nostril only, bring your awareness to the left side of your body, in particular the left hemisphere of your pelvic bowl. As you breathe into your left hemisphere, sense the energy and vitality awakening in the left side of the pelvis. Do this for as long as feels good for you.
- When you are ready to progress to the next phase of your practice, release the pressure on the right nostril. Now, using the inside of your index finger, press against the left nostril with enough pressure to block the breath, then begin to breathe into your right nostril only, bringing your attention and awareness to the right side of your body, particularly to the right hemisphere of your pelvis. Again, sense the energy and vitality awakening in the right side of the pelvis. Do this for as long as feels good for you.

- Next, move onto an alternate nostril-breathing pattern using the thumb and index finger in the same way. Pressing the thumb onto the right nostril, breathing in through the left, after your inhale (and before your exhale) block your left nostril and exhale through your right nostril. Breathe in through the right nostril, then after your inhale (and before your exhale) block your right nostril with the thumb, and breathe out through the left nostril. Continue with this breathing pattern as you draw your breath all the way deep into your pelvic bowl.
- As you do this, sense the energy of the left and right hemispheres integrating as one and sensing full vitality throughout the entire pelvic bowl. Do this for as long as feels good for you.
- Follow with some relaxed breathing and bringing awareness to the pelvic bowl, sensing the entire pelvic bowl energy and vitality.
- To finish your practice, simply thank your body and stay relaxed for as long as feels good before bringing some gentle movement back into your body and opening your eyes.

DEEP CORE BALANCING SELF-MASSAGE

- Start at the crown of your head.
- Using two fingers (middle and index finger) press firmly to massage the crown of your head in small circular motions. You should feel the skin of your crown moving in small circles, as opposed to your hand rubbing your hair. Start in a clockwise direction, and then move to an anticlockwise direction.
- Move to your forehead. Start at the hairline and use two fingers (pointer and middle finger) in a sweeping motion to draw your fingers down to the top of your nose. Then with the in-

dex and middle finger of both hands, starting in the centre of the forehead, sweep outwards towards the temples.

- With one hand, use your thumb and index finger to massage in a sweeping motion from the inner brow to the outer brow.
- Press the third eye point (between the brows) and again create small circles with the index and middle finger, using enough pressure to feel the movement of the skin, rather than the movement of the fingers on top of the skin.
- Using two hands now, place the index and middle finger of each hand on each cheek just in front of the ears. Rub your fingers upwards to the temples and downwards to the jawline.
- Using the same two fingers of each hand, begin to sweep down the jawline starting close to the ears and finishing so that your fingers meet at the chin.
- Cup your hand around your neck, sweeping from the top of the neck to the bottom of the neck with the hand wide to begin with. Then bring the fingers closer together and sweep downwards alongside the throat. Then, using the hand to gently grasp the throat, begin to wobble the throat gently from side to side, starting with the hand at the top of your throat and progressing down towards the collarbones. Be particularly gentle at the voice box.
- Using the fingers sweep the hand from the middle of the collarbones to each side.
- Using your left hand, reach to your right shoulder, pressing into the meaty part of your shoulder and massaging and releasing any tension. You may like to use a trigger point technique here, pressing the index and middle finger firmly into any point that feels particularly tender. As you do this, breathe into the muscle beneath your finger, inviting softness. Hold until you feel the muscle soften under your fingers, but for

no longer than about 30 seconds. Repeat this on the opposite side, using the opposite hand.

- Bring one hand to your breastbone, creating long sweeping motions with the palm sweeping between the breasts from the collarbones to the abdomen.
- Progress downwards to place the palm of the hand/s onto the belly. Here you can continue with your abdominal and womb massage using some of the suggestions in the Womb Massage Practice.
- Finally, if it feels comfortable, use one or two fingers or your thumb to massage your perineum and inwards of either sit bone. Small circular motions, short sweeping motions, or a simple pressure may feel good. It may also feel good to pull the muscles of the buttocks away from each other, holding a gentle stretch.

Ultimately there is no right or wrong way to do this style of massage. Experiment with what feels good for you.

DRAW ON HIGHER CONSCIOUSNESS AND EARTH ENERGY TO CREATE FROM YOUR CENTRE

This practice helps to expand your creative centre and help you tune into what aspect of your creative energy is alive right now.

- Begin with Part One of the Deep Core Connection Practice.
- Tune into the subtle movement of your deep core with your breath, and bring your awareness to your centre.
- As you breathe in and feel your diaphragm pulling air into your body, imagine that you are drawing into your body the

energy and wisdom of Higher Consciousness/Spirit/Source (whatever terminology resonates with you).

- As you breathe out, feel your breath moving across your throat and resonating against your vocal cords. Imagine taking aligned action and speaking your truth from your centre.
- Now, sense how the pelvic floor opens and softens with each breath in. As you breathe in, imagine opening your womb to draw in powerful Earth Energy and absorb the Earth's wisdom.
- As you breathe out, sense how your pelvic floor gently recoils and contracts. Imagine using this energy to create and birth all forms of creativity from your centre.
- As you breathe in and out continue with the imagery of drawing upon Higher Consciousness and Earth Wisdom by drawing it into your centre with each breath in, and creating and birthing in alignment with self with each breath out.

During this practice you may feel a new spark of creative inspiration, or receive an answer to a question that you have been asking in relation to taking aligned action. You may also sense a stronger connection to either the left or right hand side of your deep core. If you sense a more powerful connection to the left hand side of your body, this may be a message to allow time and space for creative inspiration to build. If you sense that the right hand side of your body is more awake and dominant this may be a sign to take action.

SENSUAL SELF-CONNECTION PRACTICE

Here are some beautiful movement connection practices that can help you to connect to your sensual energy. You can combine these movements with other movement practices and/or use them as the starting point for your sensual movement practice to grow from.

- Begin by laying on your back with your feet hip-distance apart and planted on the ground.
- Bring your awareness to your breath, and breathe into your pelvic bowl. Sense the energy in this space, and your connection to this space in your body.
- Begin to gently rock your pelvis forward and backward, bringing the pubic bone towards your breastbone, then tipping your tailbone towards the ground. Make this motion as fluid and as smooth as possible. Perhaps begin with a smaller range of motion, progressively creating a larger range of movement.
- In these two (2) end of range positions (an anterior pelvic tilt with the tailbone pressing toward the ground, and a posterior pelvic tilt position with the pubic bone tucked towards the breastbone) you may like to try some gentle pelvic floor contractions to increase the awareness of this space in your body, to explore how your pelvic floor contractions feel in different positions, and to increase the blood flow to this space in your body.
- Now bring your awareness to your sit bones at the base of your pelvis. Begin to create small circles with the sit bones in your preferred direction to begin with. As you bring circular motions to the right, you may like to explore your masculine energy. Sense how this expression feels in your body. As your make circular motions to the left, perhaps tune into your feminine energy and sense how this expression feels in your body. Again, make these movements as fluid and smooth as possible.
- Finally, sense into your sacrum, and its triangular shape. As you feel the sacrum pressing into the Earth beneath, imagine

the sacrum as the base of a bowl. Begin to clock around the base of the bowl, as if you're rocking the rim of this bowl on a table. Creating circular motions in one direction, making the motion as smooth and fluid as possible. You may like to imagine silk or a gentle running stream of water and its fluidity.

- As you clock around the base of your sacrum, find any points that may feel particularly 'sticky' or rigid - when/if you find a point of rigidity, spend some time focusing on this space. Breathe into the pelvic bowl as you focus on this particular range of motion, inviting smoothness and softness. Do this as many times feels good in one direction, and then taking your circles in the opposite direction.

- Again, you may like to sense your feminine energy as you clock to the left, and your masculine energy as you clock to the right.

- Now take a four-point kneeling position on the hands and knees. Begin by tilting the pelvis in the same way you did in the beginning of this practice. Start with a small range of motion, focusing on keeping the movement within the pelvis only. As you progress, take a bigger range of motion and allow that movement to resonate through the spine, neck, and head.

- Progress to circular motions of the hip, focusing on the movement of the sit bones in a circular direction.

- Next, imagine your thorax and abdomen are inside a wine barrel. Bring a circular motion to the spine arching and curling the back as if you are moving your body to press on the edges of the wine barrel.

- Imagine now closing down the side body so that the right hip draws towards the right shoulder, and then draw the left hip bone towards the left shoulder.

- As you progress through these movement patterns, continue to feel into your sensual energy. Allow the movements to progress fluidly and intuitively, knowing there is no right way to do this.

9

CLOSING

Everything that I have shared with you in this book has been derived from experiences across my lifetime. Each piece of my journey has paved another step towards finding the next. Many times along the way, I have felt truly uncomfortable. I found myself saying and feeling things that my body knew to be true, but my mind would argue that I was being ridiculous. But at every turn, and every time I challenged my mind and asked my body for the simplest truth, the ability to trust myself would embed more deeply within my cells.

Never could I have mapped out or planned this as a pathway to my own personal revelation. Never could I have imagined what I express in here to be my truth. If I read this book five years ago, I would have sworn it was written by another woman. Even when I couldn't quite comprehend my ability to communicate with spirit through honouring my body and speaking my truth, it was happening. With deep trust, continued connection, and persistent practice towards revealing your true self and honouring your nature, you too will get to go on a magnificent journey and create a centred life that feels like you.

Coming home to your body, and to your centre, is your pathway.

Your journey is yours.

Own it.

I pay my deep respect to you, for choosing to be all of you.

Comfortable in your skin, at home in your body, and centred in your truth.

With pure blessings and deep love.

Taryn

REFERENCES

Abdool, Z., Thakar,R., Sultan, A.H., & Oliver, R.S. (2011) Prospective evaluation of outcome of vaginal pessaries versus surgery in women with symptomatic pelvic organ prolapse. *International Urogynecology Journal, 22* (3). 273-278. https://doi.org/10.1007/s00192-010-1340-9

Abrams, P., Cardozo, L., Wagg, A., & Wein, A. (Eds.). (2017). *Incontinence (6th Ed)*. Bristol UK. https://www.ics.org/education/icspublications/icibooks/6thicibook

Amour, M., Smith, C.A., Steel, K.A & Macmillan, F. (2019). The effectiveness of self-care and lifestyle interventions in primary dysmenorrhea: a systematic review and meta-analysis. *BMC Complementary and Alternative Medicine, 19* (1), 22. https://doi.org/10.1186/s12906-019-2433-8

Australia. Australian Government Department of Health. (2018). *National Action Plan for Endometriosis in Australia.* https://www.health.gov.au/sites/default/files/national-action-plan-for-endometriosis.pdf

Ben-Ami, N., & Dar, G. (2018). What is the most effective verbal instruction for correctly contracting the pelvic floor muscles? *Neurology and Urodynamics, 37* (8), 290-2910. https://doi.org/10.1002/nau.23810

Brighton, J. (2019). *Beyond the Pill*. Harper Collins Publishers.

Buchsbaum, G., Duecy, E., Ker, L., Huang, L., Perevich, M., & Guzick, D. (2006). Pelvic Organ prolapse in nulliparous women and their parous sisters. *Obstetrics & Gynecology,*

108(6), 1388 – 1393. https://doi.org./10.1097/
01.AOG.0000245784.31082.ed

Butler, D., & Moseley, L. (2013). *Explain Pain* (2nd ed.). Noigroup Publications.

Coyne, K., Matza, L., & Brewster-Jordan, J. (2009) Do we have to stop again!? The impact of overactive bladder on family members. *Neurology and Urodynamics*, *28*(8), 969-975 https://doi.org/10.1002/nau.20705

Cuss, A., & Abbott, J. (2014). *Obstetrics & Gynaecology, An Evidence-Based Guide.* Churchill Livingstone.

De Albuquerque Coelho, S.C., De Castro, E.B., & Juliato, C.R.T. (2016). Female pelvic organ prolapse using pessaries: systematic review *International Urogynecology Journal, 27* (12), 1797–1803. https://doi.org/10.1007/s00192-016-2991-y

Dietz, H.P., Kamisan Atan,I., & Slita, A. (2016). Association between ICS POP-Q coordinates and translabial ultrasound findings: implications for definition of 'normal pelvic organ support'. *Ultrasounds in Obstetrics & Gynaecology, 47*(3), 363-368. https://obgyn.onlinelibrary.wiley.com/doi/epdf/10.1002/uog.14872

Dumoulin, C., Cacciari, L.P., Hay-Smith, E.J.C. (2018). Pelvic Floor Muscle Training versus no treatment, or inactive control treatment, for urinary incontinence in women, *Cochraine Database of Systematic Reviews, 10.* https://www.cochranelibrary.com/cdsr/doi/10.1002/14651858.CD005654.pub4/full

Franco., F. & Fynes. (2008). Vaginal wind – the cube pessary as a solution. *International Urogynaecology Journal (19).* 1457

Harmanli, O. (2004). POP-Q 2.0: its time has come!. *International Urogynecology Journal. 25*(4), 447-449. https://doi:10.1007/s00192-013-2252-2

Handa, V.L., & Jones, M. (2002). Do pessaries prevent the progression of pelvic organ prolapse? Do pessaries prevent the progression of pelvic organ prolapse? *International Urogynecology Journal, 13* (6). 349-351. DOI: 10.1007/s001920200078

Johannessen, H.H., Wibe, A., Stordal, A., Sandvik, L., Backe, b., & Morkved, S. (2014). Prevalence and predictors of anal incontinence during pregnancy and 1 year after delivery: a prospective cohort study. *British Journal of Obstetrics and Gynecology, 121,* 269-280. https://doi.org./10.1111/1471-0528.12438

Johnson, P., Larson, K.A., Hsu, Y., Fenner, D.E., Morgan,. D, & DeLancey, J.O.L. (2013) Self-reported natural history of recurrent prolapse among women presenting to a tertiary care center. *International Journal of Gynaecology & Obstetrics 120* (1) 53-56. https://doi:10.1016/j.ijgo.2012.07.024

Kannan, P., Cheung, K.K.,, & Lau, M.W.M. (2019). Does aerobic exercise induced-analgesia occur through hormone and inflammatory cytokine-mediated mechanisms in primary dysmenorrhea?. *Medical hypothesis, 123.* 50-54. https://doi.org/10.1016/j.mehy.2018.12.011

Krissi, H., Medina, C., & Stanton, S.L. (2003) Vaginal wind – a new pelvic symptom. *International Urogynecology Journal of Pelvic Floor Dysfunction, 14*(6). 399-402 https://doi.org/10.1007/s00192-003-1086-8

Lee, D. (2017) *Diastasis Rectus Abdominis: A Clinical Guide for Those Who Are Split Down the Middle.* Learn with Dianne Lee

Majumdar, A., Saleh, S., Hill, M., & Hill, S.R. (2013). The impact of strenuous physical activity on the development of pelvic organ prolapse. *Journal of Obstetrics and Gynaecology, 33.* 115–119. https://doi.org/10.3109/01443615.2012.721408

Nilsson, M., Lalos, A., & Lalos, O. (2009). The impact of female urinary incontinence and urgency on quality of life and partner relationship. *Neurology and Urodynamics 28* (8) 976-981. https://doi.org/10.1002/nau.20709

Nygaard I., Shaw, J., & Egger, M. (2012). Exploring the association between lifetime physical activity and pelvic floor disorders: study and design challenges. *Contemporary Clinical Trials. 33*(4), 819–827. https://doi.org/10.1016/j.cct.2012.04.001

Royal College of Obstetricians & Gynecologists. (2015). *The Management of Third and Fourth-Degree Perineal Tears.* https://www.rcog.org.uk/globalassets/documents/guidelines/gtg-29.pdf

Sung, E., Han, A., Hinrichs, T., Vorgerd, M., Manchado, C., & Platen, P. (2014). Effects of follicular versus luteal phase-based strength training in young women. *Springerplus, 3.* 668. http://www.springerplus.com/content/3/1/668

Sylvia, H. (2007) Vaginal wind – a treatment option. *International Urogynaecology Journal (18).* 703.

The American College of Obstetricians and Gynecologists. (2020). Physical Activity and Exercise During Pregnancy and the Postpartum Period. *Obstetrics & Gynecology, 135*(4), 178-188.

United States of America. American Society of Aesthetic Plastic Surgery. (2017). Cosmetic *Surgery National Data Bank Statistics.* https://www.surgery.org/sites/default/files/ASAPS-Stats2017.pdf